T0249800

Blogs and Tweets, Texting and Friending

Blogs and Tweets, Texting and Friending

Social Media and Online Professionalism in Health Care

Sandra M. DeJong, MD
Harvard Medical School
and
Cambridge Health Alliance

AMSTERDAM • BOSTON • HEIDELBERG • LONDON
NEW YORK • OXFORD • PARIS • SAN DIEGO
SAN FRANCISCO • SINGAPORE • SYDNEY • TOKYO
Academic Press is an Imprint of Elsevier

Academic Press is an imprint of Elsevier
525 B Street, Suite 1900, San Diego, CA 92101 4495, USA
32 Jamestown Road, London NW1 7BY, UK
225 Wyman Street, Waltham, MA 02451, USA

Copyright © 2014 Sandra M. DeJong. Published by Elsevier Inc. All rights
reserved.

No part of this publication may be reproduced, stored in a retrieval system,
or transmitted in any form or by any means electronic, mechanical,
photocopying, recording or otherwise without the prior written permission
of the publisher.

Permissions may be sought directly from Elsevier's Science & Technology
Rights Department in Oxford, UK: phone (+44) (0) 1865 843830;
fax (+44) (0) 1865 853333; email: permissions@elsevier.com.
Alternatively, visit the Science and Technology Books website at
www.elsevierdirect.com/rights for further information.

Notice
No responsibility is assumed by the publisher for any injury and/or
damage to persons or property as a matter of products liability, negligence
or otherwise, or from any use or operation of any methods, products,
instructions or ideas contained in the material herein. Because of rapid
advances in the medical sciences, in particular, independent verification of
diagnoses and drug dosages should be made.

British Library Cataloguing-in-Publication Data
A catalogue record for this book is available from the British Library

Library of Congress Cataloging-in-Publication Data
A catalog record for this book is available from the Library of Congress

ISBN: 978-0-12-408128-4

For information on all Academic Press publications
visit our website at elsevierdirect.com

Typeset by MPS Limited, Chennai, India
www.adi-mps.com

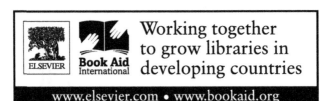

Working together
to grow libraries in
developing countries

ELSEVIER Book Aid International

www.elsevier.com • www.bookaid.org

For my family, whose love and support make
so much more possible.

Contents

Acknowledgments

As a doctor, I learn from my patients; as an educator, I learn from my students. I am grateful to the former and current child psychiatry fellows at Cambridge Health Alliance for bringing the importance of this topic to my attention and urging me to teach about it. Thanks to Cambridge Health Alliance for supporting me as a Fellow at the Harvard Macy Institute's Program for Educators in the Health Professions and to my Macy teachers and colleagues; without them, this work may never have gotten underway. Finally, I want to acknowledge my indebtedness to members of the Taskforce on Professionalism and the Internet of the American Academy of Directors of Psychiatry Residency Training: Joan Anzia, MD, Sheldon Benjamin, MD, Bob Boland, MD, Nadyah John, MD, Jim Lomax, MD, and Anthony Rostain, MD. The work we did together in developing our Curriculum on Professionalism and the Internet for psychiatry is very evident in this book; I am grateful for their wisdom. In particular, I want to thank Dr. Benjamin, my former training director, who appointed me chair of the taskforce. As a teacher and mentor, he has a wonderful quality of believing in his students more than they do in themselves.

LEGAL DISCLAIMER

Care has been taken to confirm the accuracy of the information presented and to describe emerging accepted standards. However, the author, editors, and publisher are not responsible for errors or omissions or for any consequences from application of the information in this book and make no warranty, expressed or implied, with respect to the currency, completeness, or accuracy of the contents of this publication. Application of the information in a particular situation remains the professional responsibility of the practitioner.

Introduction

A few years ago a child psychiatry fellow put in my mailbox a newspaper clipping with a Post-It note on it reading, "We should be talking more about this." The clipping was a column by Richard Friedman, MD, entitled "Take two Prozac and e-mail me in the morning" (*New York Times*, July 16, 2008). The column started me thinking about all the ways in which the digital revolution has transformed health care. In particular, I became aware of how the pillars of professionalism – boundaries, confidentiality, privacy – were being transformed by technology. I started participating in national workshops with psychiatrists and psychiatric trainees. The scope of the problem as I perceived it grew by leaps and bounds.

In 2010, a taskforce of psychiatric training directors in the United States was charged with developing a vignette-based curriculum on this topic. The demand was enormous and the response positive. When I was asked if I wanted to write a book on the topic, the need seemed clear.

But some caveats are in order: I am a medical educator, not a "techie." I am also a psychiatrist, not a nurse or a surgeon or a physical therapist. Finally, I am human, and do not have a crystal ball to see what the future may hold in terms of social media, online searching, and digital technology in health care. What follows, then, is my effort to focus on broad-based concepts of the importance of professionalism in medicine and the ways in which professionalism is at risk in the face of the scope, speed, and permanence of digital technology. I have tried to provide some context to these concepts and illustrate them with clinical vignettes. Finally, I have tried to provide both general and specific recommendations to guide health-care professionals in clinical practice as we all walk this uncharted terrain together.

I apologize in advance to those who do know a lot about technology for wherever my ignorance is in evidence. Similarly, I ask health-care professionals from other disciplines and specialties to take my vignettes with a grain of salt; they are used to make a teaching point about technology, not to reflect the reality of clinical care.

The panoply of new technological devices and innovations is more than can be fully covered in this book. Two emerging areas not included are Skype and other video-chat technologies and electronic medical records (EMRs). The former largely falls under the rubric of telemedicine and is subject to its regulations and licensing requirements. EMRs raise complicated issues for health-care facilities but largely do not involve interaction with the public except through protected portals. For these reasons, neither is addressed here.

Technology like social media and the Internet brings extraordinary opportunity to health care. How that technology is used is, at least partly, in our hands. My hope is to re-assert the professional frame in which we work and to guard the trust that our patients put in us as individual practitioners, in our hospitals and institutions, and in our profession.

Chapter | One

What is Professionalism?

The practice of medicine is an art, not a trade; a calling, not a business;
a calling in which your heart will be exercised equally with your head.

Osler, 1932, p. 368[1]

Professionalism, to paraphrase Shakespeare's Hamlet, is often noted more in the breach than in the observance. When trainees in health-care professions are asked to define professionalism, they tend to describe examples of lack of professionalism: clinicians who mistreat patients or colleagues, who put their own needs ahead of the team or the patient, who lack competence but refuse to acknowledge their limitations, and whose approach to clinical care lacks the compassion and empathy that Osler so eloquently described when he called medicine "a calling in which your heart will be exercised equally with your head" (DeJong, 2010–12). Sometimes these deficits are glaringly obvious, such as the surgeon who left the operating room to go to cash a paycheck, leaving the patient on the table (Swidey, 2004). Other times they are more implicit, only inferable by overly casual dress, sloppy documentation, poor time management, inappropriate tone of voice.

How professionalism is manifested and perceived may vary by developmental stage, gender, and geographic, ethnic and institutional cultures. Some evidence suggests that women value professionalism more than men (Roberts, Warner, Hammond, Geppert & Heinrich, 2005). Some studies suggest that views of professionalism shift over the developmental trajectory of practitioners' careers in health care (Nath, Schmidt & Gunel, 2006; Wagner, Hendrich, Moseley & Hudson, 2007). What is considered professional in one health-care

---

[1] I am indebted to Dr. Elizabeth A. Rider, who reminded me of this quotation and whose chapter "Professionalism" in Rider, Nawotniak & Smith (2007) guided my thinking about this topic.

S. deJong: Blogs and Tweets, Texting and Friending.
DOI: http://dx.doi.org/10.1016/B978-0-12-408128-4.00001-1
© 2014 S. DeJong. Published by Elsevier Inc. All rights reserved.

environment may not be in another: Jeans, open-toed shoes, and low-cut blouses may be acceptable at some institutions in some parts of the world, and within some specialties, but not in others. And culture can change over time: While scrubs used to be prohibited outside the hospital in the United States, they have now become commonplace.

But professional presentation and etiquette are not a substitute for fundamental professional attributes; the latter go deeper to the level of moral judgment, ethics, integrity, and altruism, to what Hafferty has called "the professional self":

> *Taking on the identity of a true medical professional...*
> *involves a number of value orientations, including a general*
> *commitment not only to learning and excellent of skills but*
> *also to behavior and practice that are authentically caring...*
> *There is a meaningful (and measurable) difference between*
> *being a professional and acting professionally.*
> **Hafferty, 2006, p. 2152**

The relationship between patient and health-care professional carries a "fiduciary duty": The professional has an obligation to act for the patient's benefit and the patient places ultimate faith in the abilities and good intentions of the professional. Professionalism is the foundation for the trust patients place in their caregivers. When that trust is broken, patients rightfully protest: Breaches of professionalism are a common cause for patient complaints and for negative media reports about health-care professionals (Hickson et al., 2002). In one retrospective study, physicians who were disciplined by state licensing boards were three times more likely to have shown unprofessional behavior in medical school than were those with no such disciplinary actions (Papadakis et al., 2005).

Health care has come under closer scrutiny in recent years as professionalism has been challenged by changes in health-care delivery, growing expectations by the public, the increasing role of corporate entities, and technology. The American Board of Internal Medicine (ABIM) began its Project Humanism in the 1980s and its Project Professionalism in the 1990s. Guidelines for medical schools and certification standards require demonstrated professionalism at the undergraduate and graduate level (Association of American Medical Colleges, Institute for International Medical Education, American Council for Graduate Medical Education; see Rider, 2007, p. 189). Given these requirements, efforts have been underway to try to define and assess professionalism.

In the United States, the definition of professionalism has focused more on the attributes of clinicians and their capacity to self-monitor, self-reflect, and self-regulate. Qualities such as compassion, competence, integrity, consistency, commitment, altruism, leadership, and insight come to mind (Rider, 2007). In this model, professional clinicians are those who are constantly assessing their clinical and technical skills and trying to improve; taking care of patients from the standpoint of values of humanism and empathy; shunning self-interest to focus on the care of others.

Closely related, but with a somewhat different emphasis, is the "patient-centered" professionalism model (Irvine, 2005). Writing in the UK, Irvine emphasizes the expertise of the clinician (knowledge base and skill set); the adherence to ethical virtues of beneficence, nonmaleficence, autonomy, and justice; and the service to the patient. This model reinforces the importance of developing a patient-centered health-care culture, and of a regulatory system to assess and monitor clinicians' expertise, since patients themselves are unable to do so. Implicit in this model is the notion that health-care providers should be truthful and open with their patients, and maintain patient confidentiality; they should provide patients with information so that they can make informed decisions with their providers about their care; they should acknowledge their own limitations of professional competence; and they should be respectful and unbiased towards the patient's individual and cultural values.

As Irvine's model makes clear, professionalism is often closely associated with ethics, which are typically delineated in professional codes such as the American Medical Association's code of ethics (http://bit.ly/kaaxBG). American psychiatrists Glen Gabbard and Laura Roberts have pointed out that "professionalism is embodied in ethical action" (Gabbard et al., 2012, p. 17). They emphasize the key role of biomedical ethics concepts in professional behavior (Table 1.1).

In 2002, ABIM, the American College of Physicians-American Society of Internal Medicine (ACP-ASIM), and the European Federation of Internal Medicine jointly published a document entitled, "Medical professionalism in the new millennium: A physician charter." The charter, based in part on the work of physicians Sylvia and Richard Cruess at McGill University in Canada, takes professionalism one step further to encompass not only relationships with patients, but also relationships with our students, colleagues, and society as a whole (Cruess, Johnston & Cruess, 2002). The writers argue that physicians (and arguably all health-care providers) are both healers and professionals, and that a "social contract" exists between physicians and society. This charter embodies three fundamental principles: the primacy of patient welfare; patient autonomy; and social justice. It entails ten professional responsibilities to which physicians should commit: professional competence; honesty with patients; patient confidentiality; maintaining appropriate relations with patients; improving quality of care; improving access to care; just distribution of finite resources; scientific knowledge; maintaining trust by managing conflicts of interest; and a commitment

Table 1.1 Important Principles of Medical Ethics[1]

Altruism	Acting for the good of others, without self-interest and at times requiring self-sacrifice
Autonomy	Being able to deliberate and make reasoned decisions for one's self and to act on the basis of such decisions; literally "self-rule"
Beneficence	Seeking to bring about good or benefit
Compassion	Literally, "suffering with" another person, with kindness and an active regard for his or her welfare; more closely related to empathy than to sympathy, as the latter connotes the more distanced experience of "feeling sorry for" the individual
Confidentiality	Upholding the obligation not to disclose information obtained from patients or observed about them without their permission; a privilege linked to the legal right of privacy that may at times be overridden by exceptions stipulated by law
Fidelity	Keeping promises, being truthful, and being honorable; in clinical care, the faithfulness with which a clinician commits to the duty of helping patients and acting in a manner that is in keeping with the ideals of the profession
Honesty	Conveying the truth fully, without misrepresentation through deceit, bias or omission
Integrity	Maintaining professional soundness and reliability of intention and action; a virtue literally defined as wholeness or coherence
Justice	Ensuring fairness; *distributive justice* refers to the fair and equitable distribution of resources and burden through society
Nonmaleficence	Avoiding doing harm
Respect for persons	Fully regarding and according intrinsic value to someone or something; reflected in treating another individual with genuine consideration and attentiveness to that person's life history, values and goals
Respect for the law	Acting in accordance with the laws of society
Voluntarism	Maintaining a belief or acting from one's own free will and ensuring that the belief or action is not coerced or unduly influenced by others

[1]Gabbard , G. O., Roberts, L. W., Crisp-Han, H., Ball, V., Hobday, G., & Rachal, F. (2012). Professionalism in Psychiatry (pp. 21–22). Washington, DC: American Psychiatric Press.

to these responsibilities (ABIM Foundation et al., 2002). This description of professionalism takes health-care professionals way beyond the treatment room, out into society as a whole where they have an important leadership role in advocating for quality and access, and equitable resource allocation (Table 1.2).

How do health-care professionals get into trouble with unprofessional behavior? Examples of unprofessional behavior reported by those who teach medical students and residents include dishonesty (both intellectual and personal); being arrogant, disrespectful or abrasive to the patient, students, or coworkers; failing to take responsibility

Table 1.2 Professionalism Attributes

Source	Attributes of professionalism
Accreditation Council for Graduate Medical Education (USA)[1]	Respect, compassion, integrity Responsiveness to needs of patients and society that supersedes self-interest Accountability to patients, society, and the profession Commitment to excellence and ongoing professional development Commitment to ethical principles pertaining to clinical care Confidentiality of patient information Informed consent Business practices Sensitivity and responsiveness to patients' culture, age, gender, and disabilities
General Medical Council (UK)[2]	Patient care the first concern Polite and considerate treatment of patients Respect for patients' dignity and privacy Attention to and respect for patients' views Clear communication with patients Respect for patients' right to be fully involved in decisions about their care Up-to-date professional knowledge and skills Honesty and trustworthiness Protection of confidential information Nonprejudicial treatment of patients Non-abuse of power Collegiality with peers
A Physician's Charter (ABIM, ACP-ASIM, EFIM)[3]	Professional competence Honesty with patients Patient confidentiality Maintaining appropriate relationships with patients Improving quality of care Just distribution of finite resources Scientific knowledge Maintaining trust by managing conflicts of interest Professional responsibilities

[1] www.acgme.org/outcome/comp/compFull.asp
[2] www.gmc-uk.org/guidance/archive/library/duties_of_a_doctor.asp
[3] www.abimfoundation.org/professionalism/pdf_charter/ABIM_Charter_Ins.pdf

for errors and/or not being fully invested in the clinical outcome of the patient; conflict of interest and financial gain, such as accepting kickbacks when ordering certain treatments; failure to stay up to date in clinical care; and engaging in high-risk behaviors, such as substance abuse and sexual misconduct (Duff, 2004).

While such examples clearly represent a dearth of the professionalism described in the three models above (the individual and "self-reflection," the "patient-centered," and the "social contract" models; Table 1.3), many can also be described as transgressions of implicit or explicit boundaries. The concept of boundaries implies a border or limit. *Boundary violations* occur when such borders or

Table 1.3 A Synthesis of Conceptual Models of Professionalism

Clinician's personal attributes[1]	Attributes in patient care[2]	Attributes in important relationships[3]	
		Colleagues, students	**Society**
Compassion	Strong knowledge base	Respect	Commitment to
Empathy	Expert skill	Integrity	improving health care's:
Competence	Adherence to ethical principles	Accountability	Quality
Integrity	and confidentiality	Collaboration	Access
Consistency	Respect for patient's culture	Awareness of	Distribution
Altruism	and background	boundaries	Knowledge base
Leadership	Honesty with the patient		Healer and professional
Insight	Acknowledgment of own		Management of ethical
Capacity for	limitations		principles, including
self-reflection			conflicts of interest

[1]*Rider, 2007.*
[2]*Irvine, 2005.*
[3]*ABIM Foundation et al., 2002.*

limits are crossed inappropriately, causing real or potential harm to others. *Boundary crossings* take place when the boundary is crossed but without frank harm. Sometimes, the boundary is not so clearly crossed, but rather made permeable, leaky in such a way that it becomes murky and unclear.

How does the concept of boundaries apply to professionalism and health care? First, implicit boundaries circumscribe the treatment relationship. The fiduciary relationship involves the patient placing complete confidence in the caretaker, not as a legal matter, but as a matter of the clinician's moral responsibility that comes with being a health-care professional with knowledge and training that can help the patient. When patients present for care, they are putting not only their trust but their very wellbeing into the hands of the clinician. The treatment is framed by a set of assumptions related to professionalism: the care, which will involve the patient revealing potentially highly intimate information, will be confidential; the clinician will provide a competent service; the clinician will prioritize the needs of the patient; any conflicts that the clinician has regarding the care of this patient will be directly disclosed and discussed; the clinician's role is to provide expertise and compassionate care, while the patient's role is to meet the clinician halfway and to participate in treatment decision processes.

Another set of boundaries circumscribes the health-care facilities and academic institutions in which the clinician practices. We expect, for example, that a clinician might share information with a colleague who is taking care of the patient in another service in the hospital. In fact, electronic medical records were designed in part to facilitate this process. Just as the patient may develop trust in the individual practitioner, so too may the patient learn to trust the institution as having the patient's best interests at heart.

Finally, advocates of the "social contract" concept of professionalism might argue that boundaries define the health-care profession. Society has an expectation that health-care practitioners will behave within a boundaries framework: They do the work that they do not just as a job, but rather as a calling – to do good, to help people. The assumption is that while health-care professionals may certainly charge reasonable fees, they are not primarily doing the work as a business venture. They are assumed to be solid citizens, community contributors, and individuals of moral standing. In exchange, society affords these practitioners respect, autonomy, and a voice in health care and society at large (Cruess, 2006).

A corollary to these three sets of professional boundaries, all of which involve the patient trusting their wellbeing to the clinician, the institution and the profession, is the assumption that the clinician will not take advantage of this trust. On the contrary, the clinician is expected to assume responsibility for maintaining appropriate boundaries and ensure that the patient, who is in a vulnerable and relatively disempowered position, is treated appropriately.

Unfortunately, boundary violations and crossings do occur. Sexual exploitation of patients is perhaps the most egregious. Engaging in a sexual relationship with a patient, whether it is having a sexual relationship outside the clinical setting or inappropriate sexual touching during the physical examination, sadly continues to be reported in the media. In one physician survey that found a disparity between physicians' agreements with professionalism principles and their behavior in practice, 9% of respondents reported that it was sometimes appropriate to have a sexual relationship even though the American Medical Association Code of Ethics and other standards clearly prohibit such behavior (Campbell et al., 2007). (Such hypocritical behavior has been cited as an important factor in health-care students becoming cynical about professionalism [Inui, 2003]). But there are many other ways in which a clinician can exploit the patient's dependency (Gabbard & Nadelson, 1995): Coercing the patient into certain treatments or research studies; running up unnecessary fees; scheduling of appointments to be convenient to the practitioner not the patient; accepting gifts; inserting one's own biases or values into the treatment decisions.

Of course, health-care professionals are human. Boundary crossings such as accepting hugs by patients or token gifts may be appropriate. But it is always up to the health-care professional to remain vigilant about ways in which boundaries may be eroded and what meaning boundary crossing by both clinician and patient may have in the context of a treatment relationship. Consider this example:

> *A patient who is in treatment at a medical clinic for complications from alcohol dependence is doing well, likes her treaters, and feels grateful. She starts bringing in flowers from her garden for the front desk staff and nurses, and baked goods for her primary physician. At first these gifts are only occasional. But their frequency increases to the point that at every visit, the patient is bringing in gifts. All the clinic staff members are somewhat embarrassed, but not sure what to do about them. The physician decides to explore with the patient the meaning of these gifts. Not wanting to humiliate her, he begins by thanking her for her generosity, but then underscores that gifts are not necessary: He tells her the staff has chosen to look after patients, enjoys doing the work well, and is gratified simply by getting to the know the patient and see her get better. The patient confesses that she had initially started to give the gifts as an expression of thanks. She describes herself as a "gift-giver" to her friends and acquaintances. But then, she acknowledges, she began to worry about what would happen if she stopped giving gifts. Would the staff no longer care about her? She felt that the gifts contributed to the staff's positive view of her; would she lose that? She also described needing to feel like a "good patient," just as she had always been a "good girl" and a "good student" up until the time she got into trouble with alcohol as a teenager.*
>
> Who would have guessed that these simple gifts bore such meaning for the patient? In addition, when discussing the situation with members of staff, the physician learned that they also had concerns and questions for themselves. Were the gifts making them more biased in favor of this patient? Had she become their "favorite"? Were they starting to give her extra attention because of the gifts rather than due to their own competency and professionalism? Would they start to expect that all patients would bring gifts?

This vignette illustrates how even minor boundary crossings can start to complicate and potentially compromise the treatment relationship between individual patients and providers. When frank boundary violations, such as sexual exploitation, occur, not only is the patient–provider relationship compromised but a fundamental trust in the clinician's institution and, indeed, the whole health-care profession can be brought into question or lost.

How does this discussion of professionalism and boundaries pertain to digital media and Internet technology? Technology now permeates the clinical space and is woven into the fabric of everyday lives of patients and professionals. In so doing, it has changed clinical care forever.

Clinicians and patients now have access to information about each other online that was never accessible before. As clinicians, we may not even know what patients know about us – our sexual orientation, our political affiliations, the identity of our spouses and children, the value of our home, our weekend activities, and our hobbies.

And if we become curious, we can learn the same kind of information about them.

Health-care providers have lost some of their authoritative status as health-care information becomes widely available on the Web. Patients can directly access laboratory results and other medical reports through protected patient portals. The power differential has perhaps narrowed, and care has become more collaborative. As psychiatrist and e-therapy expert Peter Yellowlees (1999) put it: "The Internet is one of the most egalitarian environments ever created" resulting in a "change in the balance of power between patients and practitioners." Perhaps because of the egalitarian nature of technology, the "Millennial" generation tends to be antihierarchical in nature, pressing for "open access" to all kinds of information previously considered proprietary, and mobilizing technology as never before, literally to revolutionize societies.

Technological innovation in general appears to be pushing conventional boundaries in new and different directions. For example, would-be authors can now self-publish online with relative ease. Scientists are bypassing government funding and going straight to "crowd-funding" on the Internet to finance research studies. Innovators talk about "pushing boundaries" and "disrupting" current paradigms. In such discussions, boundaries are portrayed as obstacles that can limit innovation as opposed to restrictions that can usefully contain behavior.

At the same time that boundaries are being challenged, information can be disseminated with the stroke of a key at any time of day and night. Its reach is wider than ever before, and can be rapidly spread, including by posting on other media. While the act of sending information is transitory, the information itself remains on servers potentially forever.

Electronic communication is not confidential: It is viewed by others (e.g., hospital IT staff, the company that owns the software), remains accessible on servers and "in the cloud," and is subject to copying and pasting, forwarding, hacking, leaking, human error, and professionalism lapses.

All of these elements of technology, and more which are discussed more deeply in the next chapter, make it a unique threat to the maintenance of professionalism and appropriate boundaries by practitioners. Professionalism breaches and boundary violations that occur by health-care professionals risk the individual's professional identity. They can lead to loss of current and future jobs, licensure, membership in professional organizations, and professional stature. But they can also damage the professional reputation of medical institutions and facilities and any academic institutions with which they are affiliated. Finally, they jeopardize that social contract which has been described as so fundamental to professionalism and risk damaging society's view of health care as a trustworthy profession.

How do we prevent professionalism and boundary breaches with technology? We teach about it. Gone are the days when professionalism was expected to be "picked up" as part of the hidden curriculum in health-care education. Given current threats to professionalism and breaches even by esteemed role models, professionalism in general and as it pertains to use of digital technology must be explicitly taught.

This book aims to do just that. It is organized into eight topics that represent potential areas of professionalism breaches online or when using digital technology. Each topic is illustrated with clinical vignettes. Most vignettes are loosely based on actual clinical stories, but are disguised. Chapter 11 spells out both general recommendations for appropriate use of digital technology in health-care practice and some specific advice for appropriate use of the different media. Finally, in Chapter 12 we will look at the road ahead for technology and health care.

REFERENCES

American Board of Internal Medicine Foundation, American College of Physicians-American Society of Internal Medicine (ACP-ASIM) Foundation, & European Federation of Internal Medicine. (2002). Medical professionalism in the new millennium: A physician charter. *Annals of Internal Medicine, 136*, 243–246. Retrieved from <http://www.abimfoundation.org/Professionalism/Physician-Charter.aspx>.

Campbell, E. G., Regan, S., Gruen, R. L., Ferris, T. G., Rao, S. R., Clearl, P. D. et al. (2007). Professionalism in medicine: Results of a national survey of physicians. *Annals of Internal Medicine, 147*(11), 795–802.

Cruess, S. R. (2006). Professionalism and medicine's social contract with society. *Clinical Orthopaedics and Related Research, 449*, 170–176.

Cruess, S. R., Johnston, S., & Cruess, R. L. (2002). Professionalism for medicine: Opportunities and obligations. *Medical Journal of Australia, 177*, 208–211.

DeJong, S. (2010–12). *"Professionalism" in administrative psychiatry seminar, child and adolescent psychiatry training program*. Cambridge, MA: Cambridge Health Alliance.

Duff, P. (2004). Teaching and assessing professionalism in medicine. *Obstetrics and Gynecology, 104*, 1362–1366.

Gabbard, G. O., Roberts, L. W., Crisp-Han, H., Ball, V., Hobday, G., & Rachal, F. (2012). *Professionalism in Psychiatry*. Washington, DC: American Psychiatric Press. (pp. 59–73).

Gabbard, G., & Nadelson, C. (1995). Professional boundaries in the physician–patient relationship. *Journal of the American Medical Association, 273*(18), 1445–1449.

Hafferty, F. W. (2006). Professionalism – the next wave. *New England Journal of Medicine, 355*, 2151–2152.

Hickson, G. B., Federspiel, C. F., Pichert, J. W., Miller, C. S., Gauld-Jaeger, J., & Bost, P. (2002). Patient complaints and malpractice risk. *Journal of the American Medical Association, 287*, 2951–2957.

Inui, T. S. (2003, February). *A flag in the wind: Educating for professionalism in medicine*. Washington, D.C.: Association of American Medical Colleges. Retrieved from <www.regenstrief.org/Members/tinui/bio/>.

Irvine, D. (2005). Patients, professionalism and revalidation. *British Medical Journal, 330*, 1265–1268.

Nath, C., Schmidt, R., & Gunel, E. (2006). Perceptions of professionalism vary most with educational rank and age. *Journal of Dental Education, 70*(8), 825–834.

Osler, W. (1932). The master words in medicine: *Aequanimitas: With other addresses to medical students, nurses and practitioners of medicine.* Philadelphia: P. Blakiston's Son.

Papadakis, M. A., Teherani, A., Banach, M. A., Knettler, T. R., Rattner, S. L., & Hodgson, C. S. (2005). Disciplinary action by medical boards and prior behavior in medical school. *New England Journal of Medicine, 353,* 2673–2682.

Rider, E. A. (2007). Competency 6: Professionalism. In A. R. Rider, R. H. Nawotniak, & G. Smith (Eds.), *A practical guide to teaching and assessing the ACGME core competencies (pp. 189–236).* Marblehead, MA: HCPro.

Roberts, L. W., Warner, T. D., Hammond, K. A., Geppert, C. M., & Heinrich, T. (2005). Becoming a good doctor: Perceived need for ethics training focused on practical and professional development topics. *Academic Psychiatry, 29*(3), 301–309.

Swidey, N. (2004). What went wrong? *The Boston Globe,* March 21.

Wagner, P., Hendrich, J., Moseley, G., & Hudson, V. (2007). Defining medical professionalism: A qualitative study. *Medical Education, 41*(3), 288–294.

Yellowlees, P. (1999). Clinical principles to guide the practice of e-therapy. In R. C. Hsiung (Ed.), *e-Therapy – case studies, guiding principles, and the clinical potential of the internet (pp. 136–149).* New York: W.W. Norton.

Chapter Two

What Makes Online and Digital Media Different?

In *Understanding Media: The Extensions of Man*, the Canadian philosopher of communication Marshall McLuhan argued that media themselves, not just the content they carry, have social implications. His popularized adage that "The medium is the message" reminds us that the medium through which we receive content deeply affects how we experience that content. McLuhan used medium, media, and technology to designate "any extension of ourselves" (1964, p. 7). One might wonder what he would have thought of the current digital revolution, the panoply of communication devices, and their respective impact on the delivery of content. In particular, we might wonder how the "media" of different electronic communications can influence our experience of the various messages in health-care settings.

Clearly, professionalism concerns such as boundaries, privacy, and confidentiality are not new. Health-care professionals have long had to contend with running into patients in the grocery store and at cocktail parties, playing multiple roles in their communities, and having the activities of their family members reflect both positively and negatively on their own professional identities. The smaller the community, the murkier the boundaries tend to be. A nurse in a pediatric office in a small town, for example, may know many of the children in the community, including much confidential information about them and their families. In the community hospital where I work, nurses, medical technicians, and interpreters often turn out to be friends or even family members of the patients. Older practitioners who have worked in these kinds of settings tend to argue that

S. deJong: Blogs and Tweets, Texting and Friending.
DOI: http://dx.doi.org/10.1016/B978-0-12-408128-4.00002-3
© 2014 S. DeJong. Published by Elsevier Inc. All rights reserved.

the Internet is no different, that these are the "same old issues" the health-care profession has been contending with for years.

And they are partially right: The underlying concepts are not that different. Before the Internet, it was still the professional's job to maintain boundaries around issues such as patient confidentiality, conflict of interest, and clinician privacy. The Healthcare Information Portability and Accountability Act (HIPAA) in the United States has underscored that responsibility. But the Internet and digital media provide opportunities for a kind of contact and communication between patients and their health-care providers that is uniquely different in several important ways. Definitions of specific digital media and their individual characteristics are given in Table 2.1.

2.1 PREVALENCE

The first distinguishing feature of the Internet and digital media is the prevalence of its use globally. Since the development of the cell phone and the personal computer in the 1970s, the convergence of ever-widening bandwidth and mobile devices with Internet capability have resulted in a "hyper-connected" world. A startling 85% of the world now has access to mobile signal. As *Nature* reported in 2009, "We've never really had a technology other than human observation that is as pervasively deployed in the world" (Kwok, 2009, p. 959). Mobile access to social media has skyrocketed. Facebook alone boasts about 900 million users, and includes about half of the population of the United States and a third of that of Europe and Australia. Over 1.5 trillion Facebook messages are sent every year (Internetworldstates.com/facebook). Even in the Middle East, where Facebook penetration is about 9%, and Africa (about 4%), the importance of social media has been dramatically evidenced in events such as the uprisings of the Arab Spring.

Internet use, at least in the United States, spans all generations. While "Millennials" (those aged 18 through 33) are more likely to go online to use social networking sites, participate in instant messaging, and read blogs, members of Generation X (aged 35–46) are more likely to go online for financial information and to visit government websites. However, certain key Internet activities are becoming more uniformly popular across all age groups, including email, online searching, and seeking health-care information. And the fastest growth in social networking is occurring in the oldest generation, aged 74 and up, whose use of social media has increased four-fold since 2008, from 4% to 16%. Similarly, searching for health information, an activity that was once the primary domain of older adults, is now the third most popular online activity for all Internet users aged 18 and older (Zickuhr, 2010).

Table 2.1 Definitions of Digital Technologies[1]

Name of technology	Definition	Use
Email	Electronic mail that may be provided by a commercial entity (e.g. G-mail from Google), or a hospital- or practice-based intranet system.	It can be encrypted to make it decipherable only to specific audiences. It can be accessed only through password-protected "portals."
Texts and Instant Messaging (IM)	Digital text or photographic messages sent via fixed-line or mobile phones and fixed or portable devices over a network, if the service plan includes it. "IM-ing" occurs in real time, and may include video.	A unique texting "language" and set of symbols has developed for texting purposes, e.g. "cul8r" means "See you later."
Search engines	Electronic searches of all online content for the search terms provided. Provided by commercial entities, e.g. Google and Bing.	Information discovered in online searches is considered in the public domain. The most frequently searched items typically move to the top of the search result list.
Social media	The general name for all interactive, web- and mobile-based technologies.	
Social networking sites	Commercial sites on which individuals may create a "page" (e.g. Facebook) or "profile" (e.g. LinkedIn) for others to search and find, thus making social and professional connections.	Settings allow restrictions on access by others. Although Facebook may be the best known, Wikipedia lists almost 200 social networking sites. Dating sites, arguably a subgroup, are not included.
Media-sharing sites	Websites for posting photographs, videos, and other media, e.g. YouTube, Vimeo.	Others can post media with content pertaining to you.
Personal webpage	A website identified by a specific domain name that can include text, photographs, videos, etc.	A professional webpage can be used for a practitioner to provide information about their practice.
Blogs	Originally "weblog," this term refers to personal web pages that typically include multiple paragraphs of content on specific subjects that is added to regularly.	Blogs can be interactive, are publicly accessible, appear on online searches, and are searchable by key terms.
Microblogs	Refers to very brief online communications, e.g. Twitter, which allows up to 140 characters per "tweet."	Messages can be sent to those who have signed on to the owner's site (as in "Follow us on Twitter") or to the public or both. Tweets are digitally archived by the Library of Congress and can be "re-tweeted" (i.e. rebroadcast to an even wider audience). Tweets can be annotated using a "hashtag" (words preceded by #).
Chat rooms	Sites on computer networks where online conversations are held in real time by a number of users.	Without video, the identity of participants in the chat room is unknown.

[1]From: 'The Ultimate Glossary: 101 Social Media Marketing Terms Explained' (now superseded by 'The Ultimate Glossary: 120 Social Media Marketing Terms Explained' available at http://blog.hubspot.com)

The prevalence of Internet and digital media use in the health-care setting is also growing. Patients expect to find medical information on the Web and discuss it with their physician by email (Baker, Wagner, Singer & Bundorf, 2003). Physicians, including psychiatrists, are increasingly using blogs and Twitter to promote their practices (Handelman, 2011; Speller & Korkosz, 2010). The Internet itself is used as a vehicle for therapeutic modalities, even to augment ongoing psychotherapeutic treatment (Yager, 2001). Social networking between patients, physicians, and other "friends" are blurring boundaries as never before (Fletcher, 2010; Gabbard, Kassaw, & Perez-Garcia, 2011; Yellowlees & Nafiz, 2010).

Increasing evidence suggests patients and physicians are communicating or having some kind of contact online and through digital media. In one survey of 4,000 physicians, approximately 20% had adopted some kind of technology (e.g. a tablet) in their practice, regardless of age or years in practice, 87% used a social media website for personal use, and 67% used a site in their professional work (QuantiaMD, 2011). In a survey of online social networking (OSN) distributed to 2,836 medical students, residents, and practicing physicians (response rate a low 16%), medical students rate of use was 93.5%, residents: 79.4%, and practitioners: 41.6%. When asked if they had visited online profiles of patients or patient family members, 2.3% of medical students, 3.9% of residents, and 15.5% of practitioners said Yes. In this same survey, 34.5% of practitioners reported that they had received friend requests from patients or their family members (Greysen, Kind & Chretien, 2010). A survey of 260 self-identified physicians on Twitter found that surgery and subspecialties represented 15% of users, internal medicine and subspecialties were 11.2%, family medicine was 9.6%, and other specialties were lower, although 26.5% fell into a category of "unspecified." The United States represented the highest area of use, with 76% of users being American. Europe was second with 5.4% and Canada third with 3.5%. Most of the public Twitter profiles contained the physician's full name and photograph and link to a website. About half were linked to a blog and only 17% to the physician's own clinical practice (Chretien, Azar & Kind, 2011).

YouTube and other video-sharing sites are increasingly used for marketing purposes and for medical specialists to network with each other. AMN Healthcare, a health-care staffing and recruitment firm based in San Diego, CA, surveyed 2,790 health-care professionals and found that 29% used YouTube for professional networking. (The most common reported medium for networking was Facebook, with 41% of responders reporting it as their first choice. LinkedIn came third with 23%.) Promotional experts report that videos allow successful "branding," and the YouTube site is easily searchable. The US Department of Health and Human Services Office of the National Coordinator for Health Information Technology has set up a YouTube channel for physicians and other health-care and information technology professionals to "share success stories and advice with physicians who may be looking for inspiration and guidance as they go through health IT implementation themselves" (Dolan, 2012, p. 1). On YouTube, physician-to-patient videos are reportedly the most common. However, some videos are clearly directed at a colleague/physician audience. Of course, all these videos can also be duplicated or posted on Facebook and blogs and linked through Twitter and other networking sites.

Unfortunately, professionalism breaches in the use of electronic and online media are also very much in evidence. In one study of medical student and resident Facebook sites, only one third of sites had appropriate privacy settings (Thompson et al., 2008). In another study of medical student deans, more than half reported having to discipline medical students for professionalism breaches online (Chretien, Greyson, Chretien & Kind, 2009). A 2010 survey of state medical boards in the United States found that 92% had received reports of online professionalism violations (Greysen, Chretien, Kind, Young & Gross, 2012). In this survey, the greatest number of violations reported occurred in the areas of inappropriate patient communication online (69%), use of Internet for inappropriate practice, including prescribing via the Internet without an existing clinical relationship (63%), and online misrepresentations of credentials (60%). A meta-analysis of weblogs by health-care professionals found nearly 17% contained enough information to identify patients (Lagu, Kaufman, Asch & Armstrong, 2008).

2.2 ACCESSIBILITY

The increased prevalence of social media and other online technologies is in no small measure due to the advent of mobile devices such as tablets and smartphones, cell phones that have Internet access; these devices are responsible for the second distinguishing feature of social media – ease of access. Half of all US adults now have a mobile web connection through either a smartphone or tablet, according to a detailed new survey of news use on mobile devices by the Pew Research Center's Project for Excellence in Journalism (PEJ) in collaboration with The Economist Group (http://www.journalism.org/analysis_report/future_mobile_news). A full 96% of 18- to 29-year-olds own a cell phone of some kind (Smith, 2010). About 75% of American teens have a cell phone and those aged 14–17 send a median number of 100 texts a day (Lenhart, 2012). In 2009–10, 89% of people in the UK had a cell phone according to the Central Survey Unit, a social survey research organization in Northern Ireland (www.csu.nisra.gov.uk).

2.3 AGGREGATING DATA AND OTHER UNIQUE PROPERTIES OF DIGITAL MEDIA

At the same time as mobile devices are expanding accessibility of digital technology, "giants" in the technology industry have started to market a full line of technology products. In an ongoing effort to garner consumer information to enhance marketing efforts, Google, Amazon, Facebook, and Apple have all expanded their products so that, increasingly, individuals' technology hardware, operating systems, browsers and navigators, email service, and social networks can all be accessed through a single provider. At ever-decreasing cost, consumers can now rent computer time and lease server space "in the cloud," such as Amazon's Elastic Compute Cloud; huge server farms are springing up across the world. Organizations are now engaging in "big data analytics," integrating data from multiple sources to identify patterns, correlations, and other useful information.

The effect of this rapidly expanding prevalence of Internet use, mobile devices, consolidation and cross-referencing of technological information is an effective shrinking of the online community. The global digital media world has become like a small village with literally millions of inhabitants. And this village is not restricted to those who actively go online and start blogging or Facebooking. Information about all of us – our political affiliations, our real estate assets, our wedding and birth announcements – is accessible online. The result is that prying, gossiping, bad-mouthing, and other negative activities renowned for occurring in small communities can and do easily happen online.

Another feature of online communication is speed of dissemination. With a click of the keyboard, digital information is transmitted globally in seconds. Email, tweets, and texts may be the most rapid but reach a more specified audience; however, that audience is quickly magnified thanks to forwarding, and copying and pasting. Media such as blogs and Facebook posts rely on people logging on; but once information is posted on these sites, depending on how privacy settings are selected, they are open to the world.

Thus, digital communication is not confidential. It is subject to forwarding, copying and pasting, hacking, leaking, human error, and professionalism lapses. Information from one individual intended for another can quickly become disseminated to the point that authorship and intended audience are lost.

Digital communication is also permanent and easily tracked. Health-care professionals who search for their name online may be horrified to see older content crop up, perhaps even postings or photographs they had hoped were long gone. The information is not limited to the professionals' own postings. Photos can be "tagged" by others, or made available by others in a whole variety of ways. According to Common Sense Media, 39% of all American teens aged 13 through 17 report posting something online that they have later regretted. At workshops on this topic, medical residents say they suspect not being granted residency positions because of online material about them. Increasingly, potential employers are performing online searches of candidates before granting interviews and jobs. A 2010 study on "Online reputation in a connected world," by a market research group called Cross-Tab, hired by Microsoft in 2009 to research online reputation information in France, Germany, the UK and the US, found that 70% of US recruiters and human resource professionals had rejected candidates based on information discovered online. The rates were somewhat lower for the UK and Germany, but the trend was the same (Cross-Tab, 2010). What kind of information has dissuaded potential employers? According to the *New York Times*, a startup called Social Intelligence surveys the Internet for everything prospective employees have said or done online over the last seven years. Information dredged up included nude photos, anti-Semitic and racist remarks, and the use of Craigslist to find OxyContin (Preston, 2011). No wonder that college students are responding by developing online reputation management services such as Brand-Yourself.com and SimpleWash (a free app for mobile phones; Kahn, 2013).

For those wishing to remove online material about themselves, the job can prove very difficult. Short of successful libel suits, anecdotal experience suggests that website owners generally will not remove content. For example, a young health-care trainee was horrified to learn that a newspaper photograph of him and his gay partner was the first item to emerge when he used Google to search for his name. He was not "out" to his patients, and asked the newspaper to remove the photo. The newspaper refused. Information stored on institutional servers may be kept for many years and is discoverable in legal actions. And even old content can be "revived" through online programs such as "The Wayback Machine." Developed by the Internet Archive, a non-profit organization, based in San Francisco, California, the Wayback Machine is a kind of digital time capsule; it allows users to see archived versions of web pages across time, which the Archive calls a "three-dimensional index" (http://en.wikipedia.org/wiki/Wayback_Machine). The creators of the service developed software to "crawl" through publicly accessible World Wide Web pages, the Gopher hierarchy, the Netnews bulletin board system, and downloadable software and collect the data which in 2009 totaled 3 petabytes (about 3 million GB). Tweets, the 140-character-maximum messages posted to followers on Twitter (which can also be "retweeted" to recipients' followers and spread rapidly to the more than 190 million users globally) are archived by the Library of Congress (Chretien, Azar, Kind, Young & Gross, 2011). The result is that, unlike bad gossip, which tends to fade from memory, information stored on the Internet lives on. As *New York Times* reporter Jeffrey Rosen (2010) suggests, "It's not just that the Web and social networking threaten your privacy. It's that there is no way in the digital age to move on, to start over – to erase your posted past" (p. 32).

The Internet and digital technology have also been an equalizing force on social hierarchies. (Recall Yellowlees' description of the Internet as "one of the most egalitarian environments ever created," 1999, p. 138.) By virtue of accessibility, portability, and the reciprocity of back-and-forth text messages, digital media erode hierarchies. For poor people living under oppressive dictatorships or "Occupy" movements, these features have proven politically powerful. They may help us understand why Malcom Gladwell and others describe the Millennial generation as emphasizing a network over a hierarchy (Scorza, 2012). The question is how this nonhierarchical culture views the traditional doctor–patient relationship. Twenty-somethings commonly address physicians by their first name, a practice that would have been considered disrespectful not long ago. As hierarchies are being challenged, appropriate boundaries are being threatened. The world of medicine is struggling with conceptualizing a doctor–patient relationship that is nonhierarchical but professional, egalitarian but mutually respectful.

Thus far, we have been focusing on broad features of social media and digital technology: widespread prevalence of use; portability and ease of access; the capacity to integrate multiple sources and create "big data;" the shrinking of the global community through digital connection; rapid dissemination; lack of confidentiality; permanence; and the antihierarchical nature of digital communication. However, how we use this technology is also important in understanding how it is changing boundaries. In part because of the advent of mobile devices, going online is no longer a "special activity" that takes place in compartmentalized space and time. Gone are the days when people have to set aside half an hour to sit down at their desk and check their email. Online technologies are accessible 24/7 across the globe, anyplace, anytime. Anyone who has walked down an urban street recently has had the experience of almost being walked into by someone who is sending a text or checking tweets on a phone. Laws have been passed to prohibit these activities while driving. Finding a restaurant, checking a fact, a spelling or a sports event score, buying shoes, and organizing a social event or a protest or streaming a video from such an event are now commonplace online activities that are integrated into the fabric of daily life.

While public online activity is in evidence everywhere, the characteristics of at-home online activity are equally important. In the privacy of one's bedroom, indeed, in bed in one's nightclothes, information can be sent digitally without the boundaried structure of being "at work" or "in the office." Adolescents are particularly notorious for going to bed with their cell phones next to them; for many people, the phone is just a reach away. How the physical and temporal context affects online communication is unclear. One might imagine, however, that the different associations to the context, the different "frame," could affect the nature of the communication, both how it is sent and how it is received and interpreted.

One of the reasons that the temporal and spatial context of digital communication may be so important is that the communication itself is currently largely restricted to text. Indeed, digital communication tends to lean towards brief, truncated textual information that relies on words and text symbols such as emoticons. Texting and tweets have almost become a language of their own in which acronyms and abbreviations become stand-ins for more precisely stated ideas: "brb" for "be right back," and "jk" for "just kidding." What is missing, besides precisely articulated words and sentences, is nonverbal clues.

Studies of human communication have suggested that up to 90% of how we communicate is nonverbal – facial expression, tone of voice, gesture and posture (Mehrabian, 1972). People with nonverbal learning disabilities or autism spectrum disorders have social deficits precisely because they are hard-wired differently and lack the ability to interpret these nonverbal cues and thus "read" people and social interactions. Even in those with high intelligence, this deficit can be highly impairing. Imagine, then, the potential misinterpretations and misunderstandings that can result from digital communication. Without the nonverbal context to provide clues about intention and meaning, emails, texts, and tweets can be experienced as angry, hostile, dismissive, removed, cold, and a whole host of other affects even when no such emotional valence was intended.

For "digital immigrants," those in the baby-boomer generation and older who did not grow up with the Internet and digital technology, all of these dimensions of digital communication are new and unfamiliar. The learning curve can be steep. As a result, digital immigrants may tend to be less facile with technology, slower to latch on to new media, and more apt to make technological mistakes. However, they may have grown up with a clearer sense of personal–professional boundaries which are expressed in a formal etiquette around communication. An email may begin, "Dear So-and-so," be written in full sentences, and "signed." Digital natives, on the other hand, grew up with digital technology. They played with their parents' cell phones as a toddler. They text rapidly and efficiently, and flit between websites, with multiple windows open on their desktop, scanning for information.

Importantly, digital natives have grown up in a world in which private and public worlds routinely intersect so that the boundaries between the two domains may to them be inherently less distinct. This phenomenon was illustrated in a workshop I co-led in which a training coordinator in a residency training program described a trainee who called in sick but when she checked her Facebook page, the trainee described being in another city visiting a friend. In the audience at this workshop was a young medical trainee, who, upon hearing this story, cried out, "That's not right. She shouldn't have looked at the Facebook page. That's private!" Older members of the audience laughed out loud, calling out how of course it was not private – information posted openly on a Facebook page was in the public domain. The generational differences in how the boundary between private and public is conceptualized were evident.

The survey by Greyson et al. substantiated this finding in American medical students, residents, and practitioners. That study found that only 45.3% of medical students and 37.4% of residents considered that online social networking activities were in a publicly viewable space. Perhaps more disturbing, only 55.6% of practitioners said they considered content on social media sites as public, suggesting a full 44.4% may view such content as private (Greysen, Kind & Chretien, 2010).

This blurring of private and public has important ramifications for professionalism on the Web, and younger generations may be particularly vulnerable to this blurring. For them, the Internet is largely an extension of their social identity. What is "self" and what is "other" can be confusing. Perhaps nowhere is this clearer than in academics and the arts. Plagiarism is on the rise, partly because the whole concept of "intellectual property" and what came from whom, when ideas or information are derived from the Web, seems to be nebulous. When a recent online novel was found to be derivative of online sources, the young author's defense was that she represents a new generation of artists who freely "mix and match media to create something new." The novel remains a best-seller and was a literary award finalist (Rosen, 2009). This topic is discussed further in Chapter 8.

In all these ways, and undoubtedly more, digital communication is markedly different from neighbors gossiping, or a doctor being witnessed a little inebriated at a Saturday-night community event, or an off-the-cuff remark about a community member who happens to be one's patient. Its extraordinary prevalence of use; portability and accessibility; capacity for "big data" analysis; tendency to shrink the global community; exponential speed and scope of dissemination; lack of confidentiality and permanence of information; dearth of nonverbal cues in all-text communications and the potential for multi-media (photographs, videos) content; the blurring between private and public, personal and professional, and self and other – all these make digital communication an inherent slippery slope for the erosion of boundaries.

In the chapters that follow, I will examine the potential impact of these specific features of digital and Internet communication on specific aspects of health-care professionalism. We will start by looking at the issue of liability and practicing according to the standard of care.

REFERENCES

Baker, L., Wagner, T. H., Singer, S., & Bundorf, M. K. (2003). Use of the internet and email for healthcare information: Results from a national survey. *Journal of the American Medical Association, 289*(18), 2400–2406.

Chretien, K. C., Azar, J., & Kind, T. (2011). Physicians on twitter. Research letter. *Journal of the American Medical Association, 35*, 566–568.

Chretien, K. C., Greysen, S. R., Chretien, J. P., & Kind, T. (2009). Online posting of unprofessional content by medical students. *Journal of the American Medical Association, 302*(12), 1309–1315. http://dx.doi.org/10.1001/jama.2009.1387.

Cross-Tab (2010). Online reputation in a connected world. Retrieved from <http://www.slideshare.net/opinionwatch/online-reputation-for-job-seekers-report-crosstab>.

Dolan, P. L. (2012). How some physicians use YouTube for networking. *American Medical News*, June 18. Retrieved from <http://www.ama-assn.org/amednews/2012/06/18/bica0618.htm>.

Fletcher, D. (2010). Facebook and how it's redefining privacy. *Time, 175*, 32–38.

Gabbard, G. O., Kassaw, K. W., & Perez-Garcia, G. (2011). Professional boundaries in the era of the Internet. *Academic Psychiatry, 35*(3), 168–174.

Greysen, S. R., Chretien, K. C., Kind, T., Young, A., & Gross, C. P. (2012). Physician violations of online professionalism and disciplinary actions: A national survey of state medical boards. Research Letter. *Journal of the American Medical Association, 307*(11), 1141–1142.

Greysen, S. R., Kind, T., & Chretien, K. C. (2010). Online professionalism and the mirror of social media. *Journal of General Internal Medicine, 25*(11), 1227–1229.

Handelman, K. (2011). ADD-ADHD Blog – The internet blog of Dr. Kenny Handelman. Retrieved from <http://www.addadhdblog.com>.

Kahn, J. P. (2013). E-trails of trouble – Young job-hunters fix online selves. *The Boston Globe*, February 14, A1, A8.

Kwok, R. (2009). Personal technology: Phoning in data. *Nature, 458*, 959–961.

Lagu, T., Kaufman, E. J., Asch, D., & Armstrong, K. (2008). Content of weblogs written by health professionals. *Journal of General Internal Medicine, 23*, 1642–1646.

Lenhart, A. (2012). *Teens, smartphones and texting*. Washington, DC: Pew Internet and American Life Project. Retrieved from <http://www.pewinternet.org/Reports/2012/Teens-and-smartphones.aspx>.

McLuhan, M. (1964, reissued 1994). *Understanding media: The extensions of man*. Cambridge, MA: MIT Press.

Mehrabian, A. U. (1972). *Nonverbal communication*. Oxford, England: Aldine-Atherton.

Preston, J. (2011). Social media history becomes a new job hurdle. *The New York Times*, July 20.

Quantia MD. (2011). Survey. Retrieved from <www.quantiamd.com>.

Rosen, C. (2009). It's not theft, it's pastiche: College students plagiarize routinely, especially from the Internet. *Wall Street Journal*, April 16. Downloaded from <http://on.wsj.com/q0DfN>.

Rosen, J. (2010). The end of forgetting, *The New York Times Magazine*, July 25, pp. 32–37, 44–45.

Scorza, J. (2012). Millennials usher in new social paradigm. Society for Human Resource Management. Retrieved from < www.shrm.org> via < http://bit. ly/SkKIBT>.

Smith, A. (2010). Mobile access 2010. Retrieved from <http://www.pewinternet. org/Reports/2010/Mobile-Access-2010.aspx>.

Speller, J. & Korkosz, T. (2010). Dr. Jeff's and Dr. Tanya's blog. Retrieved from <http://drjeffanddrtanya.typepad.com>.

Thompson, L. A., Dawson, D., Ferdig, R., Black, E. W., Boyer, J., Coutts, J., & Black, N. P. (2008). The intersection of online social networking with medical professionalism. *Journal of General Internal Medicine*, *23*, 954–957.

Yager, J. (2001). E-mail as a therapeutic adjunct in the outpatient treatment of anorexia nervosa: Illustrative case material and discussion of the issues. *International Journal of Eating Disorders*, *29*, 125–138.

Yellowlees, P. (1999). Clinical principles to guide the practice of e-therapy. In R. C. Hsiung (Ed.), *e-Therapy – Case studies, guiding principles, and the clinical potential of the Internet* (pp. 136–149). W.W. Norton.

Yellowlees, P., & Nafiz, N. (2010). Psychiatrist-patient relationship of the future: Anywhere? anytime? *Harvard Review of Psychiatry*, *18*, 96–102.

Zickuhr, K. (2010). Generations online in 2010. Pew Internet and American Life Project. Retrieved from <http://pewinternet.org/Reports/2010/Generations-2010. aspx>.

Chapter | Three

Liability, Malpractice, and Maintaining the Standard of Care

The concept of liability in medical care is rooted in professionalism and professional responsibility. In the United States, malpractice suits are considered actions in tort; i.e. a civil (noncriminal) wrong, not based on breach of contract, that has resulted in harm to someone else (Appelbaum & Gutheil, 2007, p. 115). If a health-care practitioner has established a professional relationship with a patient, the practitioner has a duty to that patient, and any proven dereliction of that duty leading directly to damage or harm in the patient may be construed in a court of law as medical malpractice. "Harm" can be either physical or emotional. An adage of forensic experts is that anyone can sue anyone for anything at any time, regardless of the merits or rationality of the case. Hence, most practitioners carry malpractice insurance, either claims-made (which is subject to lapses if the policy lapses and there is no "tail coverage") or occurrence-based (which provides coverage while the policy is in place regardless of when the claim is filed). The rising number of medical malpractice cases in the United States, and the resulting increase in malpractice insurance costs, is often cited by proponents of tort reform.

Because medical negligence cases in the United States are determined under civil law, these laws differ from state to state. However, most laws stipulate that the "duty" of the physician is to provide care and advice that meets the "standard of care." That standard is defined as care that a reasonable physician practicing under similar

S. deJong: Blogs and Tweets, Texting and Friending.
DOI: http://dx.doi.org/10.1016/B978-0-12-408128-4.00003-5
© 2014 S. DeJong. Published by Elsevier Inc. All rights reserved.

circumstances might provide. In the past, the standard of care has had a geographic parameter and was determined by the standard of the practitioner's local community. Increasingly, however, standards of care have become more consistent across the country with the advent of national association guidelines, journals, annual meetings, and continuing medical education (CME) activities (Appelbaum & Gutheil, 2007, p. 116). One might expect that national guidelines around the use of the Internet and digital technology will become part of the standard of care.

Malpractice suits are often protracted and complex proceedings. When health-care practitioners are sued for malpractice, more than one malpractice allegation is frequently made. For example, if a patient has an adverse reaction to a prescribed medication, the suit might include malpractice claims for faulty diagnosis, faulty prescribing, and faulty medication monitoring (Appelbaum & Gutheil, 2007, p. 118). The legal standard is "preponderance of the evidence." Due to difficulties in obtaining unbiased witnesses, cases often rest on what is documented in the record, and online communications about a patient are considered part of that record and are discoverable. Regardless of the outcome of such suits, the negative impact on the practitioner in terms of time, lost revenue, psychological wellbeing, and professional self-confidence can be highly significant (Menninger, Watson & Gould, 2012). If the practitioner loses the case or the case settles, results are reported to the National Practitioner Data Bank.

It is also important to recognize that even if an aggrieved patient does not file a lawsuit, the patient can still file a complaint with a state licensing board (where fitness to practice is the central concern) or the ethics committee of the relevant professional organization (where a hearing will focus on whether the standards of the organization's ethics code have been breached). In fact, as Appelbaum and Gutheil point out, patients may choose to take all three actions. Thus, possible outcomes of malpractice allegations may include not just the outcome of a lawsuit, but also everything from licensing board sanction to loss of license, and from censure to expulsion from a professional society. All these are reportable to the National Practitioner Data Bank.

One of the challenges in learning how online behaviors will be thought about by courts is that few such legal cases make their way to trial and are available as published opinions. An online search using the legal case database LexisNexis in January of 2013 found no published cases using any of the following combinations of search terms: health care or hospital or physician or doctor or medical or clinic/Internet or web or social media. A handful of ethics committee opinions from professional organizations exist and, as discussed in Chapter 1, a review of state medical boards found that of the 48 boards who responded (71% response rate), 92% had experienced at least one report of online professionalism violations. The most common (33/48, 69%) were inappropriate communications with patients online, which included sexual misconduct. Use of the Internet for inappropriate practice, such as prescribing to a patient in the absence of an established doctor–patient relationship, was reported by 30/48 (63%), and online misrepresentations of credentials by 29/48 (60%). Other infractions included breaches of confidentiality, failure to disclose conflicts of interest, derogatory comments about patients online, and online depictions of intoxication and discriminatory language. While most violations were reported by patients and their families (31/48, 65%), it is notable that 50% of the reports came from other physicians (Greysen, Chretien, Kind, Young & Gross, 2012).

While the definition of medical malpractice may seem straightforward, complexities abound. The advent of the Internet has heightened many of these complexities. This chapter will begin by outlining common areas for malpractice (some of which are covered in more detail in other chapters). It will then look at how these areas of liability can become relevant with the use of technology, and specific examples and clinical vignettes will be examined. Finally, some general suggestions to protect professionals from liability are offered.

3.1 SOME COMMON TYPES OF MALPRACTICE

3.1.1 Misdiagnosis

Patients rely on health-care professionals for correct diagnosis of their condition(s). If a health-care professional fails to recognize a condition and that failure directly causes harm to the patient and is deemed to be substandard care, the professional may be vulnerable to a malpractice claim. For mental health practitioners, failure to discern suicidality or homicidality can also fall under this category. The Federation of State Medical Boards in the USA states that a "documented patient evaluation, including history and physical evaluation adequate to establish diagnoses and identify underlying conditions and/or contra-indications to the treatment recommended/provided, must be obtained prior to providing treatment... electronically or otherwise" (FSMB, 2002, p. 5). Thus, any diagnosis made in circumstances other than face-to-face (for example, online) might open the door for liability concerns, at least for licensed physicians.

3.1.2 Negligent Use of Somatic Treatments

If diagnosis is our first job with patients, treatment is our second. Failure to meet the standard of care through surgical interventions, medications, or other treatments in such a way as to cause harm can be a liability concern. In terms of online practice, prescribing medications is obviously the greater concern: Using the wrong medication for the medical condition, not monitoring properly for side-effects, not using appropriate strategies to avoid side-effects, prescribing a medication to which the patient is allergic or for which there is some other contraindication – all can be problems in online (as well as face-to-face) prescribing practices.

3.1.3 Sexual Misconduct and Other Boundary Violations

Relationships between health-care providers and their patients are by definition intimate. The most closely held aspects of a patient's physical and emotional condition are discussed and, in the case of physical conditions, examined by intimate touching. Strong feelings can be elicited in both patient and provider, and sometimes these feelings can become sexual. A "boundary" represents the limit of acceptable behavior. Sexual contact between patient and provider is never acceptable, and crossing that boundary is a violation of the fiduciary relationship. (A chaperone is warranted during any intimate physical examination of a patient where the provider is of the opposite gender.)

Having sex online with patients is clearly not possible; however, sexual boundary crossings may be. Boundary crossings are more minor transgressions that do not result in harm to the patient. Sometimes such crossings are committed unintentionally, but can also be a conscious break from the usual frame (for example, returning the hug of a patient after her spouse has died (Gabbard et al., 2012, pp. 52–53). Boundary crossings are by definition rare occurrences. Problems may develop when they become recurrent and may act as precursors to frank boundary violations. Thus, in terms of online activity, starting a relationship with a patient through email, Twitter, texts, online dating sites, etc., can lead to a gradual erosion of boundaries, resulting in inappropriate sexual tone, word choice, and content, and ultimately face-to-face sexual encounters. A particular feature of online communication is that it is documented permanently and subject to discovery.

But even "crossings" are subject to interpretation by courts, licensing and ethics boards. As forensic experts Appelbaum and Gutheil ominously note:

> *Experience indicates that licensure boards may be especially literal-minded and even punitive in their prosecution of boundary complaints; that is they may lose the distinction between the harmless boundary crossing and the harmful*

*boundary violation. The notion of a "slippery slope,"
whereby progressive boundary incursions often end up in
sexual misconduct, becomes a "slippery cliff," whereby
even small boundary incursions (such as using the patient's
first name) are treated as though they were tantamount to
intercourse!"*

Appelbaum & Gutheil, 2007, p. 144

Other kinds of boundary violations and crossings, in addition to sexual, include other kinds of inappropriate physical contact, accepting overly generous gifts, engaging in business relationships with patients, and so on. They are all seen as potential elements in a "slippery slope," but also violations of the trust and inherent power differential between provider and patient.

3.1.4 Negligence in Supervision

With the increasing diversification of allied health professionals, as well as the extensive training required for many of the health-care professions, patients are often taken care of by someone who is supervised by someone else. That "someone else" is held liable for the acts or omissions of the supervisee. The legal doctrine in such a case is *respondeat superior* – "let the master reply" (Appelbaum & Gutheil, 2007, p.123). Thus, the onus is on the supervisor to ensure that the supervisee is performing at an acceptable standard of care. Different jurisdictions define the supervisory relationship differently. For example, in some cases an employer–employee relationship must exist; in others a consultant (whose advice may or may not be followed) is distinguished from a supervisor. How a supervisory relationship may be established online, either intentionally or otherwise, is discussed in Vignette 3.4 (p. 38).

3.1.5 Abandonment

In general, health-care providers cannot simply stop seeing patients without ensuring that their care has been appropriately transferred to another provider. But even being unavailable for a period of time can be grounds for an abandonment claim. Thus, if a patient has an emergency and the health-care provider cannot be reached and no covering provider is identified and available, then liability may be a concern. Practices that are more likely to have emergencies may have shorter acceptable response times and need tighter coverage arrangements than other, less high-acuity practices. In online practice, issues of abandonment can arise if the treatment contract either implicitly or explicitly provides for online communication but does not limit the response time or set clear procedures for what to do in an emergency.

3.1.6 Liability to Third Parties

Sometimes health-care professionals act with patients or pro-vide them with advice in a manner that can harm third parties. For example, if a patient asks for medical advice about a relative and the provider replies with specific advice, which is followed by the relative and leads to a negative outcome, third-party liability can be involved. Such advice-seeking and advice-giving can easily occur electronically.

3.1.7 Fraud

Fraud can refer to the misrepresentation of medical care in the med-ical record and medical billing. However, it can also refer to over-inflating the results that a patient can expect from a given treatment or the provider's credentials to provide such treatment, and by exten-sion the implicit expectation of success. Promises or guarantees of treatment outcomes can be made in person, but also online, either through clinical conversations through email, interactive websites, or blogs, or through online advertising. An interesting question in this era of so-called "boutique" medical practices is whether charging exorbitant fees sets up an expectation for such a high level of care that patients are at risk of being disappointed.

3.1.8 Defamation

Defamation refers to communications about a person that are harm-ful to that person. Typically, they are also false, although they may also include information that is factually true but that is deemed to have been communicated with the intent of harming the person. When defamatory comments are expressed in writing, they con-stitute libel; electronic communications fall under this category. Health-care providers need to be careful not make libelous com-ments about their patients online; such comments might include embarrassing facts, public disclosures of private information, and painting the patient in a false light. Both this and the problem of what to do if our patients make negative comments about us or reveal private information with the intent of harming our reputation are discussed in Chapters 4 and 5.

3.1.9 Breach of Privacy (including Appropriation of Identity)

This topic, which can co-occur with libel, applies when a health-care professional reveals patient-identifying information online without a patient's consent. It can include text, photographs, and videos. See Chapter 5 for an in-depth discussion.

3.1.10 Negligent Failure to Protect Patients from Harming Self or Others

While psychiatrists and other mental health professionals may deal with this topic routinely in their work with suicidal and homicidal patients, in many jurisdictions health-care professionals are mandated to report potential harm to vulnerable patients. This important topic is covered in more depth in Chapter 9.

3.2 THE DOCTOR–PATIENT RELATIONSHIP

A critical determination in any malpractice proceeding is whether the defendant did in fact hold a "duty" to the plaintiff. Other ways of asking this question are, "Was a doctor–patient relationship established?" or "Did the nature of the relationship and content of the communication between the two parties constitute medical practice?" No one is obligated to help another. A driver who comes across a car accident that has just occurred is not legally obliged to stop and help. Similarly, in most cases health-care providers are not mandated to treat every person in need of care that they happen to encounter. In fact, "Good Samaritan" laws protect the public from liability if they do stop to help someone in need, and health-care professionals have the right not to enter into treatment with people who ask for their services.

However, once a treatment relationship has been entered into, then the duty to care for the patient is established. And there lies the rub. In online communications – emails, interactive websites and blogs, Facebook sites, and other media – providers may provide medical advice to a specific patient in such a way as to inadvertently establish a professional relationship and a duty to care.

As Recupero points out (2005, p. 470), in the case of *Miller v. Sullivan* (1995)[1] a telephone conversation can be sufficient to initiate a doctor–patient relationship if "it is foreseeable that the patient would follow the doctor's advice." In this case, Miller, a dentist, telephoned his friend Sullivan, a physician, and reported symptoms of a myocardial infarction (MI). Sullivan instructed Miller to come to his office immediately, but instead Miller finished his work with patients. When he arrived at Sullivan's office several hours later, he did in fact have an MI and ultimately died. Miller's family filed a malpractice claim which was rejected by summary judgment and then appealed. The New York appellate court reaffirmed the summary judgment. However, the opinion from the court stated that, "A telephone call affirmatively advising a prospective patient to a course of treatment can constitute professional service

---

[1] 214 A.D.2d 822 (NY App. Div. 1995)

for the purpose of creating a physician–patient relationship". The court added, "it must be shown that it was foreseeable that the prospective patient would rely on the advice and that the prospective patient did in fact rely on the advice." It is not difficult to imagine a similar scenario occurring by email or text. Regardless of what the physician intends by providing advice, if the patient acts on it, a jury may find for the plaintiff if the argument that the plaintiff had the perception that he or she was in the professional's care is persuasive (Recupero, p. 470).

Another issue in the question of establishment of a doctor–patient relationship is whether such a relationship can be implicitly, rather than explicitly, established. Recupero (2005) cites the case of *Adams v. Christi Regional Medical Center*.[2] In this case, a physician provided advice by telephone to the mother of a very sick young woman. Although the medical advice was provided to a third party (the mother) rather than directly to the patient, the court ruled that the physician did have a duty to the young woman. In the judgment, the court stated that when no ongoing physician–patient relationship exists, "the physician's express *or implied* consent to advise or treat the patient is required for the relationship to come into being" [my emphasis]. In addition, the judge in this case specifically instructed the jury that "A physician–patient relationship may be created in any number of ways, including the act of a physician agreeing to give or giving advice to a patient in person *or by telephone*" [my emphasis]. Thus this case seems to set a precedent for advice by electronic communication being sufficient to create a doctor–patient relationship, even if consent for medical treatment is implicitly rather than explicitly given by the patient.

To what extent are patients requesting medical advice online from health-care professionals? One example of such electronic communication is unsolicited requests for medical advice from patients via email and interactive websites. Two studies analyzed the nature and content of such unsolicited requests. Widman and Tong (1997) looked at 70 unsolicited emails sent by patients in the course of a year in response to a website focusing on cardiac arrhythmias. They noted that 15 were questions about diagnosis, 48 about treatment, 1 about prognosis, and 6 pertained to patient education. A study of 209 emails sent to a university's dermatology department over 4 months in 1997 found that 40% of all emails could have been answered by a librarian, 27% could be appropriately responded to by a physician's email, and 27% would have required a face-to-face evaluation for a professional response (Eysenbach & Diepgen, 1999).

A number of studies have looked at what health-care professionals are doing online and whether their activity constitutes medical

---

[2] 19 P.3d 132 (Kan. 2001)

practice. Culver and colleagues examined 1,658 consecutive post-ings on an online discussion group over a 5-month period. Almost 60% of these messages were found to address a medical topic. Of these, almost 70% contained medical information, and of these mes-sages, 5.1% were authored by health-care professionals.

In 1997 and 1998, Eysenbach and Diepgen (1998a) sent an unsoli-cited email to 58 physicians and webmasters. The email, from a fict-itious patient, described an acute dermatological condition and asked for the provider's help. Fifty percent of recipients responded to the email. Of the respondents, 31% refused to give advice without having examined the patient, 59% explicitly mentioned the correct diagnosis in their response, and 17% gave treatment advice in detail, 5% includ-ing specific medications. The authors point out that the response time was highly variable, and in some cases significantly delayed (up to 10 days). The same investigators also sent a similar email to 17 "cyber-docs," 7 of whom charged for their online services and 10 of whom did not. Ten of the 17 responded and 3 declined, saying they were not experts in dermatology. Seven of the 10 who responded gave med-ical advice, 2 for free and 5 for a charge. In five cases the advice was accurate and the correct diagnosis (herpes zoster) was mentioned. The advice did not appear to meet the appropriate standard of care in two cases (Eysenbach and Diepgen, 1998b).

A similar study by Sandvik (1999) sent a fictitious email regard-ing the case of a woman with urinary incontinence to 75 websites providing information on the topic. And a 2000 study (Oyston, 2000) used an email about a fictitious patient who reported having had to be put on a breathing apparatus after a previous surgical inter-vention and who was seeking advice regarding upcoming surgery given this history. In the latter study, 54% of physicians contacted responded, 41% of whom suggested a diagnosis. In all these cases, a significant portion of physicians provided general advice online that could be construed as providing medical care.

Loyola University law professor John D. Blum (2003), an expert in health law and policy, has posited four major uses for the Internet in medicine: information; community development (among users with similar diagnoses or interests); transactional (i.e. sales of med-ical products and e-prescribing); and diagnosis or treatment pur-poses. Whether such activities constitute medical practice depends on the statutory descriptions of medicine (in the USA, outlined in each state's medical practice act), telemedicine law, and statutory interpretations of administrative and common law.

For Internet activities that involve diagnosis or treatment, med-ical boards and courts may also determine whether an online activ-ity should be construed as medical practice. In Massachusetts, for example, the Massachusetts Board of Registration in Medicine issued an opinion letter in 2003 holding that medical diagnosis provided electronically does constitute medical practice (cited in Blum, 2003, p. 42). In the case of *Wasserman v. Board of Regents of the State of New York*[3] the state court concluded that diagnosing, treating, operating or prescribing need not be limited to direct patient care, but could include preparation of medical reports and might apply to a physician administrator. In general, a connection between an online activity and an element of the legal/statutory definition of medicine would seem to suggest that such an activity would be defined as medical practice.

Two other areas of Blum's categorization of online medical activity – information and transaction – offer more of a gray zone. (The area of community development appears to be relatively free of liability concerns, unless physicians start participating in online support groups and chat rooms, intended only for patients, in a way that involves providing advice to individual patients). Providing general medical information online in a blog or on a website would be defined as e-health or telehealth rather than the practice of medicine. Again, however, the more specific and individualized the information provided, the more it may be construed as practicing medicine. (Bulkeley, 2003, details Kaiser Permanente's efforts to set up a website for diabetic patients to assist them in managing their disease.) Similarly, if physicians recommend products sold and purchased on the Internet in a general way, or sell products online with little exchange of information about the user, they are most likely not engaging in the practice of medicine. However, if they recommend specific products for specific patients following online diagnosis, then such behavior could be classified as medical practice (Blum, p. 423).

A murky area is that of prescribing and online pharmacies, an area that has come under scrutiny from professional associations and state medical boards. Legal actions against prescribers have involved practicing in a state without a license (an important risk of healthcare practice involving the Internet), or prescribing without taking a history and performing a physical. Although states differ on this subject, the American Medical Association (AMA) and the American Telemedicine Association have deemed that a face-to-face examination is necessary for prescribing, although "there are no legal specifications as to what constitutes 'face to face' or what makes up such an examination" (AMA Internet Prescribing No H-12.956 available at http://www.ama-assn.org; Linkous, undated, p. 3). In general, controlled-substance drugs can never be prescribed or dispensed over the Internet (Linkous, p. 3).

---

[3]212 NYS.2d885 App Div (1961)

The Federation of State Medical Boards documents cases of Internet prescribing violations and established a National Clearinghouse on Internet Prescribing (http://www.fsmb.org/ncip. html). For example, the Federation cites the 2002 case of a physician who was "indicted on counts of conspiracy to commit money laundering and four counts of distribution of anabolic steroids and four counts of misbranding drugs held for sale with intent to defraud and mislead" (FSMB, 2008, p. 4). The Federation also provides a listing of the specific language in each state's laws regarding Internet prescribing (FSMB, 2012). In 2008, the United States government enacted the Ryan Haight Online Pharmacy Consumer Protection Act in order to prevent the illegal sale, abuse, and trafficking of prescription drugs over the Internet (Pubic Law No 110-425, cited in Linkous, p. 2).

Digital technology easily allows for the involvement of third parties such as parents, offspring or spouses of patients. *Bienz v. Central Suffolk Hospital*[4] and *Adams v. Via Christi Regional Medical Center*[5] both involved third parties. Thus, practitioners may inadvertently establish a physician–patient relationship not just with the patient but also with those people around the patient.

In some situations, as mentioned above, the effort to help someone in distress is protected by "Good Samaritan" laws. In the United States, for example, Good Samaritan statutes provide some immunity to health-care providers who give unsolicited assistance at the scene of an accident. Thus, a bystander to an unconscious victim can provide cardiopulmonary resuscitation without worrying about liability. According to Patricia Kuszler (2000), the definition of a scene of an accident is generally narrow, and would not include responding to an email request for help.

3.3 VIGNETTES

Let us now look at specific clinical vignettes pertaining to some of the areas of liability outlined above, and the thorny question of when a treatment relationship is established.

Vignette 3.1 Misdiagnosis

A female family physician in a remote area provides practice information and general medical advice on the practice's social media site. The physician highlights clinical issues in a timely way; for example, during the summer months, advice on sun protection is posted. The physician receives a message on the site from a woman in a neighboring town who rather embarrassedly admits that she has redness and

---

[4] 163 A.D.2d 269 (NY App Div 1990)
[5] 19 P.3d 132 (Kan. 2001)

flakiness on one of her breasts. She has been so embarrassed about her condition, she has been unable to show her breast to her primary care physician, who is male. In her message to the family physician, she wonders what the condition is and what she should do about it. The physician responds saying the problem cannot be diagnosed without seeing the area of concern. The patient responds by sending the physician a photo of her right breast, which reveals redness and desquamation around the area of the right nipple. The physician responds that the lesion appears to be eczema, and recommends some topical treatments. The physician also encourages the patient to see her primary care physician. The patient dutifully applies the topical preparations but the condition does not improve. Three months later, the patient is diagnosed with Paget's disease of the breast, a malignant condition.

Was a doctor–patient relationship established in this case? Are there any liability concerns? Given that the physician responded to the woman's electronic communication with a specific diagnosis and a specific treatment, and that the patient complied with this medical advice, it would seem that a professional relationship was in fact established and that the physician now has a duty to the patient. Such a duty might involve following up on the patient's care to see if the condition is improving, or at least providing advice about what to do if the condition does not improve. The liability concerns here could include both breach of privacy if any patient-identifying content was transmitted electronically without the patient's prior consent, and misdiagnosis, which may have resulted in harm to the patient if the cancer was caught at too late a stage to be thoroughly treated.

Vignette 3.2   Negligent use of somatic treatment/ abandonment

A psychiatrist who regularly uses email with patients under the hospital's protected portal receives an email from a patient on lithium. The patient reports feeling "a little funny" as if she is "coming down with the flu." The psychiatrist emails back within 36 hours and asks the patient to say more about these symptoms. The patient emails back 24 hours later that she thinks her symptoms must be due to the fact that she has been exercising a lot in hot weather, and she is sure she will feel better tomorrow when the weather is forecast to cool off. The psychiatrist does not email back. Two days later the patient presents to the emergency room with symptoms of lithium toxicity. While in the ER she falls due to ataxia and fractures her hip.

DeJong, S. et al., 2011, Vignette #12

In this case, there is an existing treatment relationship and the physician's duty to the patient is clear. There is no breach of confidentiality because the communication occurs over a protected portal, which is encrypted and typically involves the patient signing a consent before having access to the portal. The concern here is around negligent somatic treatment. The patient is calling with symptoms that could be consistent with known side-effects of toxic levels of the medication; however, the physician tries to handle the interaction over email, not recognizing that a potential emergency is at hand. Although this failure could certainly have occurred by telephone as well, both telephone and face-to-face encounters offer more nonverbal data; for example, perhaps the psychiatrist would have heard slurred speech by telephone. Emails also leave a written record that can be presented under subpoena in court by a plaintiff's attorney.

What should the psychiatrist have done differently? Because of the potentially urgent nature of the patient's concern, the psychiatrist should have responded to the patient's first email by telephoning the patient to learn in more detail about the symptoms. If unable to assess over the telephone, the psychiatrist should have asked the patient to come in for an urgent appointment or proceed to an emergency room for evaluation. How should the psychiatrist proceed now? The risk here is that the psychiatrist may avoid contact with the patient, particularly if she feels fearful or guilty. Such a response may only make matters worse by raising potential issues of abandonment. Instead, the psychiatrist should contact her malpractice insurance carrier or the risk management department at her home institution, or both, and continue her role as outpatient psychiatrist during the hospitalization. Does the psychiatrist have any liability exposure? Yes. The psychiatrist did not meet the standard of care in recognizing the potential for lithium toxicity and addressing it adequately, and her failure to meet the standard may have led directly to the patient's hip fracture (DeJong, S. et al., 2011, Vignette #12, Teacher's version).

Vignette 3.3   Sexual misconduct/boundary violations

A young, male physical therapist is referred a middle-aged widow who is suffering from hip pain. The therapist diagnoses piriformis syndrome, and begins weekly sessions of exercises. At the first session, the therapist gives the patient his business card, which includes his email address, and urges her to contact him with any questions she has about how to do the exercises at home. The patient does have some difficulty with the exercises and so she emails the therapist to get clarification. At first the emails pertain only to her physical symptoms and the exercises. However, soon the patient is describing how helpful she is finding the sessions, and how the muscles in her buttocks and groin area are feeling much stronger. She goes on to describe that she does the exercises while she is listening to music, and asks the therapist what kind of music he likes to listen to. The therapist responds with some of his musical preferences, and describes a concert he attended over the weekend. Soon the therapist and the patient are sending several emails a day, sharing their thoughts and feelings. One day, the therapist's colleague observes him emailing on his smartphone and asks whom he is so busy emailing. When the PT tells him, the colleague raises his eyebrows and makes a facial expression that engenders concern in the therapist, and he decides to stop responding to the patient's emails.

Here again, there is an established relationship and the duty to the patient seems clear. The online communication does not seem to have occurred in the context of an ongoing informed consent discussion; thus the therapist may be vulnerable to claims of confidentiality violations. Because there is no clear harm to the patient in this case, it would be difficult to argue that malpractice has occurred. However, by engaging in personal discussion with the patient around music and other personal topics, the therapist is engaging in a boundary crossing, leaving the door open for an "inappropriate communication" allegation. The physical nature of their work together and the patient's specific mention of pelvic anatomy are potentially concerning. The patient's perceptions and psychological make-up are important to understand. If she perceives that the relationship is becoming more intimate and that the developing feelings are mutual, the therapist's abrupt cessation of contact may result in feelings of hurt and anger. There is then the risk that, particularly if she is psychologically vulnerable, the patient may displace these feelings into actions against the therapist. Such actions could include allegations of inappropriate touching, breach of confidentiality, and other boundary violations.

Vignette 3.4   Negligence in supervision

A physician maintains a medical blog that provides health information and responds to unsolicited questions. She receives a question from an early-career physician about how to manage a difficult case of a young woman with abdominal discomfort and a sensation of "fullness" despite having not eaten. The online query describes having performed multiple physical exams on the patient, all of which have been with normal limits. Nonetheless, the patient continues to report her symptoms. The young physician reports that the patient does have a history of being in psychotherapy and on psychotropic medications. The physician who authors the blog responds that given the negative work-up and the patient's psychiatric history, it is likely that the case represents a psychosomatic disorder. She recommends referral to a psychiatric consultant. The psychiatric consultant recommends an abdominal ultrasound which reveals an ovarian teratoma, which on pathological examination proves to be malignant.

This case is an example of how an online relationship can be established not only directly between a professional and a patient, but also between a supervisor and a supervisee, where the supervisee is the one with the direct relationship with the patient. This is a complicated area; however, the same standards of providing specific advice which the recipient of that advice then follows may apply. Thus, by providing advice about how to manage this specific case, this physician blogger appears to establish a supervisor–supervisee relationship, and may become liable for the patient's care. This is an example of potential liability to a third party, which is discussed further in the next vignette. By providing such advice without having ever examined the patient and by misdiagnosing the patient, the physician appears to be negligent. If the case were to go to trial, whether the patient sustained damage in this case may be decided by the make-up of the jury, the strength of the prosecution, and how sympathetic the physician blogger appears in court.

With the advent of remote supervision of all kinds of medical care from radiological findings to psychiatric diagnosis, supervisors need to be careful to define the nature of their responsibilities and their liability coverage. If frank telemedicine is being practiced in which ongoing care is provided remotely, the provider may need to be specifically licensed for this service wherever the patient resides.

Vignette 3.5   Liability to third parties

A nurse practitioner (NP) evaluates a young woman who is new to the practice. The patient has numerous, all fairly minor, medical complaints. In taking a psychosocial history, the NP learns that the young woman has a history of sexual abuse by her biological father. She spent some of her childhood in foster care, and since turning 18, has had little contact with her father. Recently, he has been trying to reconnect with his daughter, and the patient identifies this as one of the key stressors in her life. She attributes her worsening physical complaints to this stress. Concerned, the NP strongly advises the patient to maintain her distance from the father given how destabilizing his contact appears to be for her. In subsequent sessions, all scheduled to monitor the patient's physical complaints, the patient continues to describe her father's efforts to reach her, and the NP continues to advise her to keep a distance. She offers specific advice about how to reply to the father's intrusive emails and texts. In one session, the patient takes out her smartphone and shows the NP a recent text from her father. The NP takes the smartphone from the patient and texts back that he should leave the patient alone.

In this case, a third party, the patient's father, has implicitly entered the clinical space. While the NP may certainly express concern about the stress that the patient is under, providing the specific advice to avoid her father may be overreaching into the realm of undue influence. Recupero (2005, p. 471) cites the case of *Ramona v. Ramona*,[6] in which a psychotherapy patient accused her father of sexual abuse after a sodium Amytal interview. She confronted her father with these accusations at a therapy session. When the father lost his marriage and his employment, he brought suit against the therapist, and the court ruled that "therapists owe a duty to third parties to whom they direct their interventions." One might imagine such a case being extrapolated to medical encounters. In addition, by texting the father, the NP is potentially engaging in a breach of confidentiality, as well as establishing a treatment relationship without having evaluated the patient face-to-face. Care must be taken not to engage in providing even casual advice to third parties, who are often relatives of patients.

Vignette 3.6   Fraud

A health-care professional launches a website that advertises "lifestyle treatments" such as treatments for sexual dysfunction, baldness, weight loss, and smoking cessation. The website states that treatments available through the site will be "life-changing." Customers who seek services via the website can obtain prescriptions for sildenafil for sexual dysfunction, orlistat for weight loss, finasteride for hair loss, and buproprion for smoking cessation. The professional does not have personal experience in prescribing these drugs, nor any direct experience with patients in helping them with these kinds of clinical problems. The professional's credentials are not available on the site.

In this case, the website advertises that it will provide health care but it is essentially a vehicle for e-prescribing. The credentials of the person providing the "care" are not provided. In fact, this provider does not seem to be qualified to be prescribing these medications; nor does there seem to be evidence of meeting guidelines for e-prescribing (e.g. an ongoing doctor–patient relationship, follow-up arrangements, documentation in a medical record). Among the many problems in this case is fraud: The site advertises more than it delivers. The door appears to be wide open for a malpractice claim in the event of a negative outcome.

---

[6]Napa County Superior Court No. 61898.

3.4 GENERAL RECOMMENDATIONS FOR AVOIDING MALPRACTICE ONLINE

Specific recommendations for how to manage different technological and Internet media are discussed in Chapter 11. For the following discussion of clinical approaches to preventing negligence and malpractice, I am indebted to Appelbaum and Gutheil's discussion in their chapter on "Malpractice and other forms of liability" (Appelbaum & Gutheil, 2007, pp. 141–163).

Errors by health-care professionals and negative outcomes of treatment occur as part of life and human fallibility. Why, then, do some such events result in malpractice litigation (even though most do not)? Forensic experts typically say that the answer lies in the personality and psychology of the professional, the personality and psychology of the patient, and how the two people feel and behave in the context of a bad outcome. Depending on these factors, any intervention or treatment that results in harm to the patient can result in patients feeling shock, anger, and betrayal. The professional is also likely to have strong feelings, including shock, fear, anger, and guilt. Both the patient and the physician are at risk of acting out on those feelings: The patient may launch various forms of attack, including legal action, and the professional may engage in defensive behaviors such as avoidance. A downward spiral may develop in which, for example, the professional's avoidance (perhaps being unresponsive to the patient's email and phone calls) may heighten the patient's feelings of abandonment and resulting anger. Patients and physicians who are psychologically vulnerable – e.g. those suffering from personality disorders – may be increasingly at risk in situations of bad outcomes. One study of false sexual misconduct allegations in psychiatric practice found that more than 90% of the cases could be attributed to patients with borderline personality pathology (Gutheil, 1985).

Two mainstays of protection are maintaining a high standard of care and a strong doctor–patient relationship. If these are evident in the medical record and in how the professional presents in court, the professional may be adequately protected. The former is beyond the scope of this book. The latter brings us back to Chapter 1 and the importance of maintaining professional behavior. What kinds of behaviors in the professional relationship are most helpful in protecting us from malpractice and negligence?

First, the professional needs to recall the ethical principles of beneficence and nonmaleficence and the duty to act in a manner that helps rather than harms the patient. Indeed, the patient's needs must come first (the principle of fidelity). To this end, professionals must take care not to exploit patients and to avoid the appearance of exploitation. As discussed above in the section on "Sexual misconduct and other boundary violations," boundary crossings and boundary violations involve crossing an implicit line from professional behavior, in which the patient's needs are first, to unprofessional behavior, in which the provider's needs are put first. Most obviously, these transgressions can be sexual. However, any alterations in the frame of practice (seeing the patient in one's home, providing care in a sidewalk conversation) can be viewed this way.

Financial boundary crossings may occur if a patient accepts monetary gifts from the professional, or vice versa, or if the professional exploits his or her professional status and position of power with the patient to financial gain. A physician who has shares in a medical device company, and who then encourages a patient to use the services of that company by sending the patient promotional emails, may be perceived as coercive, even if the potential conflict of interest is disclosed. A relationship in which the professional fosters an overly dependent relationship with the patient, including frequent online check-ins that exceed the clinical indication, is another example.

Of course, sometimes unintentional boundary crossings occur. For example, a treater and patient may discover that they are both "friends" on the same Facebook site. These kinds of boundary crossings are best addressed promptly and explicitly, including an exploration of the patient's feelings about the situation and how to proceed. The discussion should be documented appropriately in the record.

Avoiding abandonment is important. Perceived abandonment is a crisis for the patient and likely to generate strong feelings. One way to avoid abandonment is to maintain an open-door policy (Appelbaum & Gutheil, 2007, p. 145): According to such a policy, a patient who is being treated by a provider is always welcome to return. Of course, practitioners may feel that they can no longer work with the patient: If the patient has not paid their bills, is pursuing legal action, has been physically threatening, or even simply if the practitioner feels unable to do any more to help the patient, the practitioner may choose to refer the patient to another qualified and available provider. Note that such a transfer of care cannot ethically occur in the context of a clinical emergency.

Similarly, practitioners should take great care with the issue of covering their practice when they are not available. All electronic media used to interface with patients need to make clear if a practitioner is unavailable and what the coverage arrangements are. Illness is an important example. If out of the office due to illness or medical procedures, health-care professionals should obtain coverage, and not try to take care of patients while they are also taking care of themselves.

Practitioners should limit their practice to the treatment of patients and medical conditions they are qualified to treat. For example, providing online advice to children when one is only qualified to treat adults raises concerns. One of the challenges with unsolicited emails and interactive websites is that the treater may not know how old the patient is.

Voicing an apology when a professionalism breach has occurred can be very healing, and in some jurisdictions treaters who do so are protected under the law. For example, in Massachusetts, physicians who apologize for a regrettable action are protected by a law which states that such apologies are "inadmissible as evidence of an admission of a liability in a civil action." Small transgressions can occur relatively frequently. For example, if a physician who routinely uses email with patients inadvertently sends an email to an incorrect address, the best approach is to admit the mistake, apologize, and talk through the repercussions with the patient. Such apologies also help to set a frame of respect for the patient and attention to aspects of professional practice.

Showing respect for the patient is another key ingredient to a strong doctor–patient relationship; for instance, by calling the patient by the correct name (always starting with the more formal), being punctual or offering an apology for lateness, focusing on the patient during discussions and avoiding distractions like the laptop and electronic medical record. Online manifestations of respect are often conveyed through the elements of "netiquette" – appropriate word choice, tone, structure, and content (see Chapter 10).

In practical terms, preventing malpractice often involves setting the frame ahead of time. Applying this concept to technology might mean having a privacy notice with patients that clearly delineates the routine use of technology in the practice (for example, how information is stored and secured, who in the office will have access to the information). Rather than advertising services that cannot be safely or consistently provided, the limitations of such use should be emphasized. If specific electronic media are to be used, providing written informed consent, and making informed consent an ongoing process in the treatment, is a way of explicitly acknowledging the risks and ensuring that the benefits perceived by the patient continue to outweigh them. This can be a tricky area for technology: While open communication often greatly enhances clinical treatment, patients' judgment can also be compromised due to illness, time pressures, anxiety, and eagerness to please the treater. The treater must take the initiative to re-assert the frame and remind the patient that all communication should occur in a way that feels appropriate to the patient.

Providing specific advice to patients online or otherwise is another complicated area. In general, making any treatment a shared decision between provider and patient is preferable to a paternalistic approach in which the providers act as if they know better. Patients can push us in this regard, and we may feel compelled. But unless a competent patient waives the right to an informed consent, we should avoid making treatment decisions without them. And if patients ask our advice on personal matters, caution is warranted. Is direct advice ever warranted? Certainly in the case of an emergency, or with a patient who is so emotionally compromised or regressed as to be unable to make a decision, such an action may be appropriate.

When patients do act out on their feelings in inappropriate ways or start to talk about seeking legal action, providers would do well to stay calm and not engage in arguments with the patient. While they should probably seek their own legal counsel, practitioners may also want to think about what feelings the patient is acting out on and respond accordingly. For example, if a patient is feeling humiliated, an acknowledgment and apology may be appropriate. Above all, practitioners need to avoid seeing the patient as an aggressor and themselves as the victim; such a frame is likely to result in negative acting-out behaviors.

The AMA guidelines on Internet use admit that Internet prescribing can provide a useful service (from http://www.ama-assn.org). The effort is to establish good uses of the Internet for prescribing while state medical boards pursue unprofessional prescribing behaviors. In addition to requiring an examination prior to online prescribing, the guidelines emphasize the need for a thorough informed consent, arrangements for follow-up care, sending prescriptions to pharmacies over a secure network (e.g. AMA Internet ID), including the prescription in the medical record, and providing physician-identifying information. Exceptions include consultation, in which another provider will follow up with the patient, and on-call coverage where access to the medical record is available (American Medical News, 2003).

The issue of prescribing medications online or discussing somatic treatments via electronic means raises a couple of additional concerns. One is if the medication could impair the patient's functioning. The issue of prescriber liability for patients doing harm to others allegedly due to the effects of a medication is an emerging liability area. In such cases, the patient commits the negligent act that harms, but if the prescriber did not duly warn the patient of the potential for such behavior and document that warning (perhaps a recommendation not to drive at all), the prescriber may be at risk of malpractice allegations. Similarly, medications that can be abused, stolen, or re-sold may pose an additional risk to the patient. Electronic communication can be helpful if such concerns are appropriately documented, but is an additional liability if such documentation is absent.

This brings us to the discussion of documentation as a whole. When providing treatment, a clinician must document the decision-making process. First is the risk–benefit analysis, which outlines alternatives to treatment (including the option of no treatment). Second is the clinical thought process that went into the decision. For example, a prescriber might recommend a medication with a longer half life over one with a shorter half life if compliance with medication has been a past impediment to effective treatment for this patient. Third is documentation of the patient's capacity to engage in decision-making about the treatment.

Other aspects of documentation are facts, judgments, and reflections. Documenting the process of treatment provides protection for the health-care professional in court, and failure to do so opens the door for malpractice or negligence claims. Critical events and acts should be recorded. Response and impediments to treatment should also be recorded. Emergencies require particularly careful documentation. The practitioner's thought process, decision-making, and evidence used (including consultation) should be included. If suits are threatened, this too needs to be documented, as does consultation with risk management staff. As with all documentation, medical records should be written in a professional manner.

All electronic communication that documents medical decision-making and practice should be included in the medical record, with appropriate labeling, such as patient's name and date of birth. Communication that contains an error or professionalism breach should be appropriately corrected without attempting to alter the existing record. The exact timing of electronic documentation is easily determined; thus, any effort to retrospectively alter a record is largely futile and casts a defendant in a suspicious light.

In addition to documentation, a second "leg" of a practical approach to malpractice prevention is consultation. Consultation is distinct from supervision in that a consultant is brought in to a case previously unfamiliar to him or her and asked to provide advice without assuming any responsibility for the patient's care. Consultation can be on an "as-needed" basis, or a more regular arrangement in which a senior colleague or a group of peers provides input on cases. Electronic communication has facilitated consultation in certain ways, by providing a quick way to inform consultants of clinical questions as well as a text record of the discussion. However, the same concerns about confidentiality breaches as in other forms of communication exist, and email consultation should probably be discussed in informed consents with patients. In addition, the speed of electronic communication may mean that health-care providers are quick to respond to patients' direct questions before seeking consultation about issues which may be beyond their expertise or comfort level. Consultation about technology itself is often indicated and needs also to be documented in the record.

If a patient does file a lawsuit against a health-care provider, the provider should not drop out of contact or refuse to communicate with the patient. Such an approach invites additional allegations of abandonment. Rather, the provider should proceed as a professional clinician, thinking with the patient about how best to proceed, assisting in finding alternate care, and working with risk management and legal experts to develop a plan of action.

CONCLUSION

In summary, medical practice involving electronic media harbors many of the same liability risks as regular face-to-face medical care: misdiagnosis, negligent use of somatic treatments, sexual activity with patients and other boundary violations, negligence in supervision, abandonment, liability to third parties, fraud, breach of confidentiality, and defamation. The particular characteristics of Internet and digital media can make some of these potential problems an even greater concern for providers. In order to prevent malpractice and negligence allegations, providers would do well to maintain a high standard of care and protect the doctor–patient relationship and the treatment alliance, including avoiding inadvertently entering a treatment relationship. Establishing a clear treatment frame, being scrupulous about maintaining complete and accurate documentation, and obtaining and documenting ongoing consultation are all mainstays of a practical approach to malpractice prevention.

ACKNOWLEDGMENTS

I am indebted to Paul S. Appelbaum and Thomas G. Gutheil for their excellent chapter, "Malpractice and other forms of liability" in Appelbaum & Gutheil, 2007, for content related to and organization of this topic. I would also like to thank Megan Hayes, Esq., for assistance in conducting online research of legal cases.

REFERENCES

American Medical News Editorial, (2003). Web prescribing: How to set the standards. Amednews.com. Retrieved from <www.ama-assn.org> via <http://bit.ly/176e6T9>.

Appelbaum, P. S., & Gutheil, T. G. (2007). *Clinical handbook of psychiatry and the law*. Philadelphia, PA: Wolters Kluwer/Lippincott Williams & Wilkins.

Blum, J. D. (2003). Internet medicine and the evolving legal status of the physician-patient relationship. *Journal of Legal Medicine*, 24(4), 413–455.

Bulkeley, W.M. (2003). Diabetes website to provide customized treatment plans, *Wall Street Journal*, May 14.

DeJong, S. et al. (2011). Curriculum on professionalism and the Internet in psychiatry. Retrieved from <www.aadprt.org> via <http://bit.ly/Yh1JRq>.

Eysenbach, G., & Diepgen, T. L. (1998a). Responses to unsolicited e-mail requests for medical advice on the World Wide Web. *Journal of the American Medical Association, 280*(15), 1333–1335.

Eysenbach, G., & Diepgen, T. L. (1998b). Evaluation of cyberdocs. *Lancet, 352*(9139), 1526. http://dx.doi.org/10.1016/S0140-6736(05)60334-0.

Eysenbach, G., & Diepgen, T. L. (1999). Patients looking for information on the Internet and seeking teleadvice: Motivation, expectations, and misconceptions as expressed in e-mails sent to physicians. *Archives of Dermatology, 135*(2), 151–156.

Federation of State Medical Boards (2008). Internet prescribing table. Retrieved from <www.fsmb.org/pdf/internet_prescribing_table.pdf>.

Federation of State Medical Boards (2012). Internet prescribing – Law and policy language (by state). Retrieved from <http://www.fsmb.org/pdf/InternetPrescribing-law&policylanguage.pdf>.

Gabbard, G. O., Roberts, L. W., Crisp-Han, H., Ball, V., Hobday, G., & Rachal, F. (2012). *Professionalism in psychiatry*. Washington, DC: American Psychiatric Press.

Greysen, R. S., Chretien, K. C., Kind, T., Young, A., & Gross, C. P. (2012). Research Letter: Physician violations of online professionalism and disciplinary actions: A national survey of state medical boards. *Journal of the American Medical Association, 307*, 1141–1142.

Gutheil, T. G. (1985). Medicolegal pitfalls in the treatment of borderline patients. *American Journal of Psychiatry, 142*, 9–14.

Linkous, J.D. (undated). The Challenge of regulating internet prescribing. Retrieved from <www.americantelemed.org> via <http://bit.ly/XJOx9g>.

Menninger, E., Watson, N., & Gould, D. (December 1, 2012). *The personal experience of being sued. Physicians and healthcare professionals in court: A survival guide.* Boston, MA: CME Course, Harvard Medical School/Beth Israel Deaconess Medical Center/CRICO/Risk Management Foundation.

Oyston, J. (2000). Anesthesiologists' responses to an email request for advice from an unknown patient. *Journal of Medical Internet Research, 2*, e16.

Recupero, P. R. (2005). E-mail and the psychiatrist–patient relationship. *Journal of the American Academy of Psychiatry and the Law, 33*(4), 465–475.

Sandvik, H. (1999). Health information and interaction on the internet: A survey of female urinary incontinence. *British Medical Journal, 319*(7201), 29–32.

Widman, L. L., & Tong, D. A. (1997). Requests for medical advice from patients and families to health care providers who publish on the World Wide Web. *Archives of Internal Medicine, 157*(2), 209–212.

Chapter Four

Confidentiality

Confidentiality and privacy, as we will discuss further in Chapter 5, are similar but not the same. Confidentiality pertains to a particular status that can be given to information or data indicating that it "is sensitive for some reason, and therefore … needs to be protected against theft, disclosure, or improper use, or both, and must be disseminated only to authorized individuals or organizations with a need to know" (American Society for Testing and Materials, cited in Buckovich, Rippen & Rozen, 1999, p. 123). Confidential information is typically only disclosed in a relationship of trust, with the assurance and expectation that the information will not be shared. A "confidentiality agreement" details what information may be made available to those who have been authorized to receive it. Usually such authorization is given by the person the information is about (Nelson, 2011, p. 2). Thus, patients or their guardians seeing a health-care provider may sign authorization forms to release confidential medical information to others involved in their care.

Privacy, on the other hand, relates to the person and has to do with a broader right to freedom from unwanted intrusion. It applies to everyone, including both patients and health-care professionals. An implicit zone of privacy protects individuals' personal lives and personal information. Where the precise boundaries of that zone are drawn varies between individuals and cultures. As treaters we are given the patient's implicit or explicit permission to step into that zone and perform intimate physical examinations and ask about details of their personal life. This is part of the fiduciary relationship: Our patients trust us not to violate their privacy by keeping information about them confidential, and it is our moral duty to respect that trust. A more utilitarian approach to confidentiality is that if we did not respect patients' confidentiality, they would not disclose

S. deJong: Blogs and Tweets, Texting and Friending.
DOI: http://dx.doi.org/10.1016/B978-0-12-408128-4.00004-7
© 2014 S. DeJong. Published by Elsevier Inc. All rights reserved.

important information to us and our capacity to diagnose accurately would be jeopardized, in turn potentially jeopardizing the public health (Appelbaum and Gutheil, 2007, p. 4.)

Of course, in everyday life, we can ask that information be kept confidential by those to whom we disclose it; in health care, the confidentiality of patient information is protected under the law. It is worth noting that the same is not true for health-care practitioners; in this way, confidentiality may be distinguished from privacy in health care: Patients are free to talk about us with others, say things about us online, and reveal the content of appointments with us. We are not free to do the same about them. One may wish that patients would not disclose private information that they happen to learn about us out of a sense of respect for our privacy, but patients do not have a legal obligation to protect our privacy in the same way that we are legally obliged to protect theirs by keeping information confidential.

In the United States, the confidentiality of patient information is protected under the Health Insurance Portability and Accountability Act of 1996 (HIPAA), Public Law 104-191. Sections 261 through 264 of the Act require the Secretary of Health and Human Services to publish standards for the electronic exchange, privacy, and security of health information. The final version of these standards, which govern "individually identifiable health information," were published some years later and became known as the "Privacy Rule" (HHS, 2002). The rule applies to health-care providers "regardless of size, who electronically transmit health information in connection with certain transactions [including] claims, benefit eligibility inquiries, [and] referral authorization requests." The patient information, termed "protected health information" (PHI), must be protected regardless of how it is transmitted – electronically, on paper, or orally. HIPAA sets a minimum expectation for protection of confidential information. Other federal laws, state laws, and statutes, as well as institutional or licensing regulations, may set higher standards that can take precedence. For example, according to the U.S. Federal Alcohol and Drug Treatment Confidentiality law, disclosure or redisclosure of a patient's participation in a substance abuse treatment program that is federally assisted is illegal without a signed consent (http://www.samhsa.gov/healthprivacy/docs/ehr-faqs.pdf).

Although patients and practitioners may feel burdened by an increase in privacy paperwork, the alleged intent of HIPAA was not to be purely restrictive. Rather, a major goal was to assure that individuals' health information is properly protected while allowing the flow of such information in order to provide and promote high-quality health care and to protect the public's health and wellbeing. The rule strikes a balance that permits important uses of information, but at the same time protects the privacy of people who seek care and healing (http://1.usa.gov/4K3FbJ, p. 1 of Summary of the HIPAA Privacy Rule).

In practice what this means is that the release of any information about a patient must be authorized through a consent form signed by the patient. The release should specify the type of communication (e.g. telephone, release of records), the type of information to be released, for what purpose, and the time frame to which the release applies. For technological communication such as email, the potential risks and benefits of the communication, including potential breaches of confidentiality, need to be made explicit (see Chapter 11). For some jurisdictions and patient populations, as indicated above, particularly sensitive health-care information may require specific consent. According to the final version of HIPAA that goes into effect in September, 2013, as well as the HITECH Act that was passed as part of the 2009 American Recovery and Reinvestment Act, HIPAA-covered practices will need to give patients privacy notices that include breach avoidance and notification procedures (including for breaches by subcontractors), conduct security risk assessments, and be prepared to give patients copies of their electronic records (Lubell, 2013).

As discussed in Chapter 1, confidentiality has long been a standard of professionalism. It is core to the notion of the fiduciary relationship. Because of the nature of the work that we do, we elicit from patients and they tell us extraordinarily intimate information. Some of that information is verbal – how they feel, stressors they are encountering, specific symptoms about various parts of their body, details of their personal and family histories. An important part of the information is nonverbal, transmitted through: tone of voice, gesture, expression; physical findings on examination; results derived from various tests and sample-taking from their body. In some areas of health care such as surgery, patients literally open themselves up to us while they themselves are unconscious. This is perhaps the greatest act of trust.

4.1 CONFIDENTIALITY, SOCIAL MEDIA, AND THE INTERNET

Violations of confidentiality in health care are not new. Hallway and elevator conversations about patients have been unfortunately common. The particular features of digital technology and the Internet, however, make confidentiality a particularly sensitive and vulnerable issue in health care. First, electronically transmitted information is – almost by definition – not confidential. It is viewed by information technology personnel at institutions; by employees of software and technology hardware companies; and by the increasing array of companies whose servers are leased for the storage of information.

Recently, industry leaders in technology have promoted the idea that information can be stored "in the cloud," suggesting that it is far away and accessible from anywhere. A "cloud" is in fact a physical server located on one of the growing number of huge server farms across the world (Dolan, 2013; Glanz, 2012).

Not only is the information generated by any one individual on the Internet not confidential, but technology offers the capacity to exponentially increase the size of the intended audience with extraordinary speed. A message that was intended for a small group of people can reach the mobile devices and computers of literally thousands of people in seconds. This power of technology has been harnessed in fascinating and new ways, from social uprisings like the 2011 Arab Spring to the organization of flash mobs at Grand Central Station. Finally, because it is stored on servers, electronic information is largely permanent and always revocable; errors are not easy to erase. When this scope, speed, and permanence are applied to a breach of confidentiality, the effects can be devastating to patients and their families, health-care practitioners, the institution in which they practice, and, indeed, to health care as a profession.

How do online and electronic confidentiality breaches occur? Some occur in a manner beyond the practitioner's control, as in hacking, viruses, or cutting, pasting, and forwarding of content. Others happen intentionally through practitioner bad judgment, thoughtlessness, and venting. These will be discussed through examples.

On April 22, 2010, the following item appeared in the police blotter of the *Needham Times*, a community newspaper in the town of Needham, Massachusetts:

A Needham psychological therapist reported on April 13 that someone hacked into her e-mail account and sent messages to her clients telling them she was in trouble, police said. The woman reportedly told police she received a phone call from a client asking her if she was in any trouble. She reportedly told the client she was fine. The client reportedly said she received an e-mail from her saying she was in trouble in Spain and if she could send her money. The woman received several other similar phone calls from concerned clients and friends. Later, when the woman tried to access her Yahoo account, she was reportedly unable to log on. After contacting Yahoo, she was reportedly told someone apparently hacked into her computer and sent out the distress e-mails using her e-mail account. Yahoo was reportedly able to make her computer functional again, but the victim reportedly lost about a thousand contacts from her e-mail account.

Needham Times, p. 8

Since this story appeared, a very similar story has been described by others in various media. A random hacker was apparently able to access the psychologist's contact list, which includes the names of her professional clients – clearly patient-identifying information. This is likely a case of a "black hat hacker," someone who chooses to hack out of maliciousness or personal gain (see Hacking 101 tutorial at http://bit.ly/fOWWd8). Hackers may choose targets for an underlying reason or randomly.

Hackers can access secure networks in a variety of ways. "Vulnerability scanners" are tools that allow hackers to quickly scan a computer and identify security weaknesses. "Password cracking" is a system that allows hackers entry to secure sites by obtaining the password. A "rootkit" allows a hacker to hide the hacking. Some information is obtained by hackers through "social engineering," a practice that involves in some way posing as the owner/user of the secure system and pretending to be having access difficulties. Skillful hackers can use such tactics as intimidation, name-dropping (to elicit a sense of false confidence in IT personnel), and taking advantage of a help desk staff member's inclination to want to be helpful, in order to get required information.

Sometimes hackers will use a "Trojan horse," a computer program that looks like it is doing one thing but is actually doing another, in order to obtain future "backdoor" access to a computer. Viruses are self-replicating programs that work by being inserted into existing code or documents; when a user mobilizes this code or document, the virus is propagated. A "worm" is similar, but does not need to insert itself into a program or be mobilized by the user in order to replicate. Any of these hacking tools can result in the unintended, rapid spread of confidential content on the Internet.

Another kind of unintended dissemination of confidential information electronically occurs with human intervention: Virtually anything posted electronically can be copy and pasted and disseminated through additional means, or can be forwarded using the technology on which the posting was originally sent. Emails, tweets, blogs – all are subject to this potential magnification, literally within seconds. Often the duplication and forwarding process is not malicious in intent; but the result can be the widespread dissemination of what should have been confidential material. Consider an email, for example, from one medical colleague to another seeking help with a complicated case. The email is initially sent within the firewall of the hospital's intranet. (Firewalls are not impermeable, but they are currently the best protection we have to reduce electronic permeability.) The email contains specific information about the patient which would not make her recognizable to the general public, but potentially recognizable to anyone who knew her. The colleague who receives the email is not sure about the best answer to the clinical questions posed, and so forwards it to a colleague at another institution asking for help. That person in turn forwards it to another expert, who actually recognizes the patient as someone who had previously been in his practice.

While the confidentiality breaches described above cannot be blamed on the person who originally wrote the electronic message, other breaches are well within that individual's control. This is where professionalism can play such an important role. Bad judgment, poor use of humor, thoughtlessness, and venting can all contribute to the dissemination of confidential information online.

One example of this kind of unprofessional behavior online that jeopardizes patient confidentiality is a 2006 study of healthcare blogs (Lagu, Kaufman, Asch & Armstrong, 2008). The authors defined medical blogs as those that contained some medical content and which seemed to be written by physicians or nurses. Blogs were identified by a Google search using the term "medical blog." Two hundred and seventy-one medical blogs were identified, all the blogs were reviewed, and content was categorized. The blogs were written in the first person like a journal. In some cases, the blogger was explicitly identified; in others, the blogging was done under a pseudonym (e.g. pandabearmd.com). Of these, 56.8% contained enough information to identify the blogger, and 42.1% contained information about patients. In almost 18% of these blogs, patients were described in negative terms. Of the blogs that described interactions with individual patients, almost 17% provided enough detail to enable the patient to be recognized. In three blogs, photographs of the patients were posted. Such cases reflect poor judgment by people who had apparently not read the Healthcare Blogger Code of Ethics (available from http://medbloggercode.com/the-code/).

Sometimes the confidentiality breaches are more malevolent than in the cases we have discussed so far. Consider the following example:

> Dr. A, a psychiatry resident leaving his on-call shift in the emergency room at a local hospital, decides to send his friends a Facebook update. "Just finished with a lousy 24-year-old jerk," Dr A writes. "A soldier complaining of pain = addict." Dr. B, who is an emergency medicine resident in the same local hospital and Dr A's Facebook friend, sees the status update on his smartphone just before going in to see a 24-year-old male patient with a military history who is complaining of pain.
>
> **DeJong et al., 2011, Vignette #31**

Here, an undoubtedly exhausted resident leaving his shift loaded with complicated feelings towards his most recent patient interaction chooses to vent online using his Facebook page. In a large, urban community, the odds of two physicians seeing the same patient on the same night might be remote. However, at a community hospital, the odds suddenly become much higher. Thus, what may not have been "patient-identifying information" in HIPAA terms in the larger setting becomes it in the smaller. The impact of this particular breach may have been relatively minor in terms of the dissemination of confidential material. But one would imagine that the ER physician enters the room with preformed biases against the patient. And the negative venting by the psychiatry resident, which would presumably be viewed by others, reflects badly not only on that individual, but on psychiatry and the medical profession as a whole.

Strong feelings frequently result in the loss of good judgment. When we are sad, angry, overwhelmed, frustrated, or resentful, we may post content that we would not consider posting when in a calmer state of mind. We are more vulnerable when we feel unsupported and alone. Imagine, for example, leaving a hard day on a medical inpatient service. A patient you have cared for has just died despite your best efforts. You disagreed with the recommendations of a subspecialist involved in the patient's care, but deferred to that specialist. You feel depleted and cope by posting on your Facebook page what a bad day it has been and why, and you criticize the handling of the case by the subspecialist in sufficient detail that the identity of the patient could be inferred by anyone who had worked on the same service. Such behavior could constitute an HIPAA violation and a breach of professionalism. You would have done better to consult a peer or a supervisor and talk through the difficult feelings around the case.

Sometimes bad judgment is masked as humorous content. What can seem humorous to one person, or in one particular moment, can quickly become not so funny to another person or in a different time or context. For example, young health-care workers may think it fun to post pictures of themselves and their friends looking silly while intoxicated on their Facebook page. However, when a supervisor or prospective employer sees that content, the lack of professionalism will be evident and may have dire consequences.

Posting online comments about patients under a pseudonym does not protect us from HIPAA violations. Online postings can be traced, to the chagrin of one Boston pediatrician who blogged about a malpractice case in which he was the defendant. When the plaintiff's attorney asked the pediatrician in court whether he blogged under the pseudonym "The Flea," the case quickly settled (Cooney, 2007).

Mobile devices have greatly heightened the risk of confidentiality breaches. Because smartphones combine cameras with Internet access, health-care professionals have been able to take photographs and videos of patients and disseminate them on the Internet, for example on their Facebook page. As a result we have seen headlines in the media such as "Nurses fired over cell phone photos of patient – Case referred to FBI for possible HIPAA violations" (WISN, 2009) and "Posting of brain photo on Facebook sparks inquiry at Syracuse's Upstate Medical University" (Mulder, 2009). Even benign content like pictures of patients' babies should probably not be taken and should certainly not be disseminated electronically.

Sometimes, confidential information is disseminated by the patients themselves. For example, a 1994 study of email communication between patients and their physicians found that 90% of patients relayed important and sensitive information electronically (Neill, Mainous, Clark & Hagen, 1994).

What is the impact of such confidentiality breaches? Unfortunately, the potential impact is broad and largely negative. Such breaches create a rupture in a professional health-care relationship. If patients discover breaches, they may feel violated and as a result become angry and vengeful. If they continue in treatment with the professional, the atmosphere can be one of distrust. They may hold back information. If the treatment relationship falls apart, patients may file complaints with hospital grievance officers, licensing boards, or ethics committees of professional organizations, or file malpractice lawsuits.

For the practitioner, the consequences can be severe. An HIPAA violation can result in a significant fine to the provider and to the institution. The practitioner can lose his or her job, license, and membership in professional organizations (Greysen, Chretien, Kind, Young & Gross, 2012). For example, a Rhode Island physician was fired from her job at Westerly Hospital after she vented about a patient on her Facebook page. Although the patient's name was never mentioned, the hospital stated that enough details were reported to identify the patient. The Rhode Island medical board subsequently reprimanded the physician and fined her $500 (Conaboy, 2011). That particular story was reported prominently in the *Boston Globe* and the Rhode Island newspapers. Undoubtedly, public opinion of that particular physician and perhaps the hospital that had hired her was negatively influenced as a result. In fact, seeing such stories of professionalism violations in the media has become commonplace. The net effect is to cast the whole health-care profession in a negative light. The very tenets of professionalism, discussed in Chapter 1, appear to be violated by such behavior.

4.2 VIGNETTES

Let us now turn to some more examples of how confidentiality can be violated in online behaviors and digital communication.

Vignette 4.1

After being discharged from an inpatient service, a female patient Googles the name of one of the male nursing staff recently responsible for her hospital care. She finds the nurse "cute" and hopes to invite him out on a date. The second item on the search list is a link to the nurse's blog. While reading the blog, the patient feels some of the content is about her. The blog refers to a "20-something blond with an attitude and an a___ to go with it," and other details about this individual's presentation and care. The patient is hurt and angry. She calls the hospital grievance officer with a complaint about confidentiality.

Adapted from DeJong et al., 2011, Vignette #30

Are there any confidentiality issues? If it is deemed that enough identifying information is in the blog to identify the patient, the nurse may have violated HIPAA and may be fined, fired, and otherwise sanctioned. This vignette exemplifies the considerable risks of discussing our professional care of any individual patient online. What makes matters worse in this case is the negative content about the patient. It may be the insult, particularly in light of the patient's attraction to the nurse, which resulted in the call to the grievance officer. The trust she had placed in the nurse had been violated. If the patient had contacted the nurse directly with her complaint, he might have had the opportunity to do a repair, to apologize, to reassure her that he was talking about someone else, or to acknowledge that the behavior was reprehensible. Once the complaint had gone to administration or to a licensing board or ethics committee, a process began to unfold and the matter was out of the nurse's hands. Thus, it is the feelings elicited in the patients as much as the professionals' actions themselves which can result in negative outcomes.

Vignette 4.2

A student in respiratory therapy who has just rotated off a medical service looks up the blog of one of the service physicians whom she particularly admires. The physician is a person of considerable stature in his field, and the blog provides both health-care information and some philosophical musings about the current state of health care, clinical practice, and the art of medicine. One part of the blog discusses managing "the difficult patient," and cites specific clinical examples. The respiratory therapist recognizes one of the examples as a very challenging patient whom the medical team recently discharged from the service. Although the patient's name is not used, the student is able to identify the patient by descriptors that are used in the blog.

This example raises the issue of confidentiality in an academic and teaching context. Health-care professionals often teach about their areas of expertise and in doing so draw upon clinical cases. In the past, such cases have been "disguised" so as to prevent revealing the patient's identity. However, "disguising" is a subjective judgment. The current standard for publication about patients is to obtain patient consent (Snider, 1997). What should the respiratory therapist do? Certain professional guidelines do mandate that health-care professionals report to professional associations and licensing boards any violations of professionalism standards online (see Federation of State Medical Boards, Inc., 2002). The respiratory therapist would do well to consult with a supervisor or the privacy/compliance officer of the hospital to think through how best to proceed. Although such an approach may elicit anxiety on the part of the respiratory therapist, in particular because of the difference in standing between the therapist and the attending physician, the patient's right to confidentiality needs to come first.

Vignette 4.3

A pediatrician routinely communicates with her adolescent patients on her smartphone. The pediatrician believes that using smartphone technology (texts, tweets) enhances communication with these patients who are often reticent to contact her using more traditional means such as office telephone and pager. The phone is password protected, but the pediatrician's children know the password because they often use the smartphone to play games on. One day at home, the pediatrician hears her adolescent daughter squeal out, "Oh, my God! Susie has chlamydia!!" The adolescent had gone on her mother's cell phone to play games and had discovered a text exchange between her mother and an adolescent patient.

Mobile devices are particularly vulnerable to breaches of confidentiality. Technology exists to encrypt smartphone communications and separate personal from professional portals. However, not all health-care professional who use smartphones in their work employ such technologies. If the pediatrician did not have an informed consent from the patient's guardian and an assent from the adolescent to use smartphones for communication, the pediatrician may be vulnerable in this case to charges of a confidentiality breach. If the patient is a school peer or acquaintance of the pediatrician's daughter, the leak of the very personal information about the chlamydia diagnosis creates a difficult situation. Does the pediatrician just ask her daughter to keep the information confidential? What if the daughter does not? Does the pediatrician disclose the leak to her patient and patient's guardian? The pediatrician is now in a quandary that might have been prevented by keeping her password confidential, using encryption software, and using separate devices or portals for professional and personal use.

4.3 GENERAL RECOMMENDATIONS FOR PROTECTING CONFIDENTIAL INFORMATION

How can health-care professionals avoid breaches of confidentiality? Specific mechanisms for protecting confidentiality with various technologies will be discussed in Chapter 11. For now, let us focus on broad principles and underlying concepts.

An important underlying principle is the difference between public and private. In presenting about professionalism and the Internet to young trainees from across the country, I have witnessed them expressing shock and horror at the notion that a supervisor or hospital administrator would check online for information about them. Recall the medical resident who was horrified upon hearing the story of a training administrator who looked on his Facebook page after a trainee called in sick for the day. The administrator learned that the trainee had headed to the city for the day; "But that's private!" the medical resident protested.

The anecdote suggests a blurring and, unfortunately, a frequent misunderstanding about what information is public and what is private. Information posted online and unprotected by privacy walls (such as the privacy settings on Facebook) is by definition in the public domain; it can be accessed by anyone with Internet access. The administrator did not breach confidentiality nor invade the resident's privacy by looking up his Facebook page. (A more complicated question is whether there is any obligation to let someone know of your intent to look up online content about them; see Chapter 5.) Much information that was always in the public domain – marriage certificates, bankruptcy filings, court proceedings, family lineage – are now still in the public domain but are made much more accessible by Internet technology. Thus, the very concept of privacy is changing. As health-care professionals, we now must assume that patients, colleagues, and employers all can and will access private information about us online.

As much as possible, we need to separate the personal from the professional domains. For example, we might cautiously use Facebook or other social media sites in our personal lives with maximum privacy settings, but use Linked In or Doximity for our professional interactions. (Bear in mind that patients can also be on professional social media sites, so the need for judicious posting of any content does not disappear by using a professional social medium.) We might have a medical blog, but use it only to disseminate accurate and important information rather than providing any details about particular patients. We might use one email address for our work with patients, a different email address for our private contacts, and perhaps a third for any online purchases.

We need to pause before sending any information about patients electronically. Is there an appropriate signed release from the patient in place? Is there a better way to send the information? Is the content appropriate? Has the recipient's contact information been verified? Is the urge to send the content coming from negative feelings, a need to vent? Or is the urge to send coming from a place not in the patient's best interest, for example to make others laugh?

If health-care professionals choose to use electronic communication, they need to know how to use the technological devices competently. Accidental forwarding, cc'ing, and clicking on the wrong name in a global address list all happen. Similarly, practitioners need to have appropriate security software on whatever devices they use and update them regularly. Hacking and viruses can lead to the inadvertent release of patient information. Developing close relations with a trusted information technology professional can be important.

When in doubt, don't use electronic information to send information. Schedule a face-to-face meeting or a telephone call instead. In general, sensitive or complex information is never best sent electronically and can be misconstrued.

With many digital technologies, we may not know for sure who is on the other end of the communication. We can be "friended" by imposters, receive emails from those who falsely identify themselves, and be in chat rooms with users who don't identify themselves at all. Having some method for authentication can be vital. Electronic signatures and digital certificates of authenticity can help ensure the author and sender are who they appear to be (http://www.gpo.gov/authentication).

What is our obligation if we see someone else's HIPAA violation? Many medical facilities, academic institutions, licensing boards, and professional associations require that violations of HIPAA and patient confidentiality in general be reported to officials such as privacy officers and board chairs. Part of the trust that society places in us as professionals is that we will perform due diligence in monitoring ourselves. When we fail to do that, we risk losing public trust.

CONCLUSION

Confidentiality pertains to certain information that holds a special status owing to its sensitivity and the consequent need for it to be secure from disclosure or improper use. Confidential information revealed in the context of a treatment relationship should be disclosed to a third party only with the written consent of the patient or in situations where knowledge of the information is necessary to provide medical care. In the United States, the confidential status of health-care information is protected under the law by both federal standards, such as HIPAA, and potentially higher standards of state and other jurisdictions.

Confidentiality is a mainstay of professionalism. While confidentiality breaches are not new, digital technology and the Internet provide means for the rapid, widespread, and permanent dissemination of private information either intentionally (through hacking, forwarding, and cutting/pasting) or inadvertently through bad judgment and human error. Sometimes, patients themselves disclose information unadvisedly. The rise of mobile devices has heightened the risk of confidentiality breaches. Negative consequences include feelings of betrayal and anger on the part of the patient, and fines, loss of employment, and even loss of license for practitioners. In many settings, reporting the confidentiality breaches of other health-care practitioners is required.

Strategies such as clearly delineating between public and private electronic communication channels, pausing before sending information, ensuring to whom and from whom information is being sent, and being competent in the use of technology are all important safeguards again breaches of confidentiality and resulting lapses in professionalism standards.

REFERENCES

American Society for Testing and Materials Committee E31 on Healthcare Informatics, Subcommittee E31.17 on Privacy, Confidentiality and Access. (1997). *Standard guidelines for confidentiality, privacy, access and data security principles for health information including computer-based patient records*. Philadelphia, PA: AST, 2. Publication no. E1869-97. Cited in Buckovich, Rippen & Rosen (1997).

Appelbaum, P. S., & Gutheil, T. G. (2007). *Clinical handbook of psychiatry and the law*. Philadelphia, PA: Wolters Kluwer/Lippincott Williams & Wilkins.

Buckovich, S. A., Rippen, H. E., & Rozen, M. J. (1999). Driving toward guiding principles: A goal for privacy, confidentiality, and security of health information. *Journal of the American Medical Informatics Association, 6*, 122–133. http://dx.doi.org/10.1135/jamia.1999.0060122.

Conaboy, C. (2011). For doctors, social media a tricky case. *The Boston Globe*, April 20. Retrieved from <www.boston.com> via <http://bo.st/hDIdRO>.

Cooney, E. (2007). Flea's fall sobering for bloggers. *The Boston Globe*, May 21. <www.boston.com/yourlife/health/blog/2007/05/fleas_fall_sobe.html>.

DeJong, S. et al. (2011). Curriculum on professionalism and the Internet in psychiatry. Retrieved from <www.aadprt.org via http://bit.ly/Yh1JRq>.

Dolan, P. L. (2013). Cloud-based EHRs create medical privacy risks. *American Medical News,* January 14. Retrieved from <www.ama-assn.org> via <http://bit.ly/10tUHMi>.

Federation of State Medical Boards, Inc. (FSMB). (2002). Model guidelines for the appropriate use of the Internet in medical practice. Retrieved from <http://www.fsmb.org/pdf/2002_grpol_use_of_internet.pdf>.

Glanz, G. (2012). Power, pollution and the Internet. *The New York Times*, September 22. Retrieved from <www.nytimes.com> via <http://nyti.ms/102w4zy>.

Greysen, R. S., Chretien, K. C., Kind, T., Young, A., & Gross, C. P. (2012). Research letter: Physician violations of online professionalism and disciplinary actions: A national survey of state medical boards. *Journal of the American Medical Association, 307*, 1141–1142.

HHS. (2002). US Department of Health and Human Services. *Summary of the Privacy Rule*. Retrieved from <www.hhs.gov> via <http://1.usa. gov/4K3FbJ>.

Lagu, T., Kaufman, E. J., Asch, D. A., & Armstrong, K. (2008). Content of weblogs written by health professionals. *Journal of General Internal Medicine, 23*, 1642–1646. http://dx.doi.org/10.1007/s11606-008-0726-6.

Lubell, J. (2013). HIPAA gets tougher on physicians. *American Medical News,* February 4. Retrieved from <www.ama-assn.org> via <http://bit.ly/WvZFqf>.

Mulder, J.T. (2009). Posting of brain photo on Facebook sparks inquiry at Syracuse's Upstate Medical University. *The Post-Standard*, September 24.

Needham Times. (2010). Community safety – Therapist's computer hacked. *Needham Times*, April 22, p. 8.

Neill, R. A., Mainous, A. G., Clark, J. R., & Hagen, M. D. (1994). The utility of electronic mail as a medium for patient-physician communication. *Archives of Family Medicine*, *3*, 268–271.

Nelson, K. (2011). Confidentiality vs privacy. Inpropriapersona.com. Retrieved from <http://inpropriapersona.com/confidentiality-vs-privacy/>.

Snider, D. E. (1997). Patient consent for publication and the health of the public. *Journal of the American Medical Association*, *278*, 624–626.

WISN.com (2009). Nurses fired over cell phone photos of patient – Case referred to FBI for possible HIPAA violations. Retrieved from <www.wisn.com> via <http://bit.ly/XJ3jvm>.

Chapter Five

Patient and Practitioner Privacy

Like it or not, much of our personal life is no longer private. Patients can find all kinds of information about us online: where we live, the value of our home, our political affiliations, our activity on dating sites, the deaths and marriages of our family members, our children's activities. Online searching has become such an integral part of our culture, it has entered popular fiction. Pulitzer Prize-winning novelist Jennifer Egan, for example, describes the internal thought process of a young woman character in psychotherapy as she muses about her psychotherapist:

> *He wore funky sweaters and let her call him Coz, but he was old school and inscrutable, to the point where Sasha couldn't tell if he was gay or straight, if he'd written famous books, or if (as she sometimes suspected) he was one of those escaped cons who impersonated surgeons and wind up leaving their operating tools inside people's skulls. Of course, these questions could have been resolved on Google in less than a minute, but they were useful questions (according to Coz), and so far, Sasha had resisted.*
>
> **Egan, 2010, p. 4**

As a result, we should no longer be surprised when our patients google us; on the contrary, we should expect it. However, we are still human and will inevitably have feelings about it when we learn that a patient has done this. Sometimes we will learn directly from the patient about information acquired on the Internet. However, often patients will simply act in a way that reflects what they have learned. If a patient starts to behave differently towards us, we may need to consider the possibility they have learned something about us that they are having difficulty integrating into their relationship with us.

61

S. deJong: Blogs and Tweets, Texting and Friending.
DOI: http://dx.doi.org/10.1016/B978-0-12-408128-4.00005-9
© 2014 S. DeJong. Published by Elsevier Inc. All rights reserved.

If a patient brings information into a treatment session that they have learned about us online, we need to be prepared to deal with it.

This chapter will begin by looking at the concept of privacy and how much private information is available about us on the Web and is brought into our work. It will go on to examine privacy issues raised by technology for both health-care providers and their patients in a treatment setting. Finally, specific vignettes pertaining to privacy will be examined and thoughts about how to manage privacy issues will be offered.

What is privacy? In this age of paparazzi and aggressive media pursuit of celebrity news (consider the phone-hacking scandal in Rupert Murdoch's newspaper syndicate, http://nbcnews.to/TsPfnG), privacy advocates have highlighted the extent to which privacy appears to be violated in current culture. Ellen Alderman and Caroline Kennedy, for example, discuss urine toxic screening for job applicants, hotel surveillance cameras, and strip searches for traffic violations (cited in Malamud Smith, 2003, p. 5). The implication seems to be that privacy has always been a natural right. But as Janna Malamud Smith points out in her book *Private Matters – In Defense of the Personal Life* (Malamud Smith, 2003), privacy is a relatively new entitlement, perhaps a product of relative affluence and the rise of individuality; prior to a few centuries ago, communal living and shared physical space and information were more normative.

What has changed with technology is the intimate nature of the information that can be obtained and transmitted online. (As discussed in Chapter 2, all information online can be transmitted widely, quickly, and permanently.) A recent example highlights this issue: A group of scientists at the Whitehead Institute for Biomedical Research in Cambridge, MA, went online to see if they could identify people who had anonymously provided genetic samples for research. The research database was publicly accessible so that other researchers could make scientific use of the genetic data. Sure enough, using Internet searches and free, publicly accessible genealogy websites, the Cambridge group was able to identify almost 50 people (Gymrek, McGuire, Golan, Halperin & Erlich, 2013; Johnson, 2013).

As discussed in Chapter 4 (see p. 47), privacy and confidentiality are similar but not the same. Confidentiality refers to the status that can be given to sensitive information or data that needs to be protected from unauthorized access or disclosure. Sharing of such information is usually subject to a confidentiality agreement, typically authorized by the owner of that information (Nelson, 2011, p. 2).

Privacy, on the other hand, pertains to all aspects of a person, and not just information about them. Although the Fourth Amendment protects against "unreasonable searches and seizures" by the government, privacy's broader legal basis was first delineated in a seminal law review article on the right to privacy by Samuel Warren and Louis

Brandeis in 1890. They were primarily addressing the issue of secret photography. The late Alan F. Westin, Professor Emeritus of Public Law at Columbia University, expanded the definition of privacy in his landmark book *Privacy and Freedom* (1968) by describing it as our ability to control how, when, and how much information about ourselves is revealed to others, arguing that such privacy enables freedom. In so doing, Westin paved the way for the current debate around privacy and the Internet. In Westin's obituary his colleague Jeffrey Rosen, Professor of Law at George Washington University, noted that "[Westin] recognized that the problems of protecting privacy are now so daunting that they can't be dealt with by law alone, but require a mix of legal, social and technological solutions" (Fox, 2013).

Privacy relates to the notion of boundaries that we discussed earlier (see p. 5). Westin outlines four core concepts to privacy: solitude, anonymity, reserve, and intimacy (Westin, 1968, p. 31). These concepts all imply a boundary that protects from outside intrusion; the first three circumscribe a boundary of privacy around the individual and the last around a relationship. Forensic psychiatrists Appelbaum and Gutheil (2007, p. 4) describe privacy as having four basic components: "guaranteeing freedom from intrusion on seclusion; appropriation of one's name or likeness for commercial purposes; publicity given to one's personal life, and publicity that places one in a false light."

But even these conceptual frameworks leave many questions unanswered: What is an acceptable limit of other people's knowledge about us? Is the answer to that question purely an individual right? How far can and should we go in seeking information about others before being, and being perceived as, intrusive?

A key challenge is that the definition of privacy itself seems to be changing, in no small measure due to the advent of technology. As *Time* magazine reporter Dan Fletcher wrote in his 2010 cover story on how Facebook is redefining privacy: "Getting to the point where so many of us are comfortable living so much of our life on Facebook represents a tremendous cultural shift, particularly since 28% of the site's users are older than 34 ... Facebook has changed our social DNA, making us more accustomed to openness" (Fletcher, 2010, p. 33). Other cultural factors – such as reality TV, shows like Oprah Winfrey's "bare-all" approach to interviews, the celebrity gossip industry – have contributed to a shift in how much information we are comfortable with others knowing.

How has privacy been defined in the health-care context? The American Society for Testing and Materials' Committee on Healthcare Informatics defined privacy as:

> *The* right of individuals *[emphasis added] to be left alone*
> *and to be protected against physical or psychological*

invasion or the misuse of their property. It includes freedom from intrusion or observation into one's private affairs, the right to maintain control over certain personal information, and the freedom to act without outside interference.

Buckovich, Rippen, & Rozen, 1999, p. 123

This definition was adopted by American Medical Informatics Association.

Partners Healthcare, Inc., a multi-hospital health-care system in Boston, posts a document on privacy for human subjects in research in which privacy is described as the ability of an individual or group to seclude themselves or information about themselves and thereby reveal themselves selectively. The boundaries and content of what is considered private differ among cultures and individuals, but share basic common themes. Privacy is sometimes related to anonymity, the wish to remain unnoticed or unidentified in the public realm. When something is private to a person, it usually means that it is considered inherently special or personally sensitive. The degree to which private information is exposed, therefore, depends on how the public will receive this information, which differs between places and over time. Privacy can be seen as an aspect of security – one in which trade-offs between the interests of one group and another can become particularly clear (Partners Healthcare, undated, p. 1).

The statement goes on to point out that privacy refers to persons and their ability and interest to control "the access of others to themselves" (Partners Healthcare, undated, p. 1). Privacy can include the patient controlling where and when they give information, what kind of information they give, the kind of experiences the patient receives, and who will acquire and can use the information. Thus, a patient may not want to be seen entering an abortion clinic or a substance abuse treatment facility for fear of stigmatization. (Being "seen" on a chat room or website about sensitive medical conditions might be considered an equivalent kind of exposure and a reason why patients go online anonymously.)

Individuals differ in what they view as private depending on factors such as education, ethnicity, personality, and relationship with the clinician. These issues are highlighted in a 2008 study at Johns Hopkins University of privacy concerns in patients and guardians of patients with genetic and nongenetic medical conditions. In the study, 541 adults or parents of children with sickle cell disease and cystic fibrosis (genetic disorders) and diabetes and HIV (nongenetic disorders), as well as adults with or at risk for breast cancer or colon cancer, were interviewed about the positive or negative consequences of disclosure of their condition. About one-third of respondents described themselves as "private," another third as "open," and the remaining third as "neutral." Those with HIV and those more at risk for colon cancer were more likely to call themselves private than those with cystic fibrosis. African-Americans were nearly twice as likely as whites to say they were private. Having a genetic condition was not significantly related to whether patients described themselves as private. Almost all the patients said others knew about their condition, varying from spouses (99%) to friends and neighbors (47%). Overall, 74% were glad and 13% regretted that others knew about their condition. The findings were no different between the two populations (genetic vs. nongenetic). Eighteen percent expressed the hope that others would not find out about their medical condition. In spite of the generally positive feeling about disclosure, many patients had experienced discrimination in getting health insurance (27%) or employment (19%) because of their health condition (Kass et al., 2004, pp. 267–268).

As the Partners statement suggests, protecting the privacy of one group or individual can sometimes be in conflict with other interests. For example, if a family member who is diagnosed with a genetic disorder chooses not to disclose the finding to other members of the family, those family members' interests may be compromised. The cost of protecting the privacy of individual subjects in research may have the effect of lowering research participation and raising study duration and costs due to restrictions on recruitment (Harris, Levy & Teschke, 2008).

Regulating privacy has proved a difficult task, as the history of Facebook and its privacy settings have shown (Fletcher, 2010; Steyer, 2012, pp. 53–55). Europe and Britain began with a more restrictive approach: In 1995 the European Union enacted the Data Privacy Directive requiring that all 15 member countries establish national privacy laws by October 1998 (Bukovich, Rippen & Rozen, 1999, p. 122). Databases for which privacy intrusions were a risk were required to obtain licenses (Perritt, n.d., p. 2). In the United States, a more open approach was initially adopted until concerns about online privacy and "data mining" were raised (see, for example, Fienberg, 2006). In 2010, Google was fined for collecting personal information from unencrypted wireless routers as Google employees drove around neighborhoods accruing photographs and other data for their Street View mapping. In 2011, both Apple and Sony got into trouble, Apple for using iPhones and iPads to collect data about location and personal movements of users, and Sony for a breach of personal data when their Playstation network was hacked. Also in 2011, the Federal Trade Commission sanctioned Facebook for repeatedly violating privacy (Steyer, 2012, pp. 58–61). In 2013, the smartphone manufacturer HTC settled a case in which security flaws could allow users' location to be tracked without their permission and private information stolen. Hackers had easy access to install software that could send a text and record the user's phone calls. Lesley Fair, a senior lawyer for the Federal Trade Commission, who initiated the lawsuit, is cited in *The New York Times* as blogging:

> The analogy isn't exact, but it's like giving a friend the combination to a safe only to find out he's handing it over to anyone who asks ... HTC didn't test the software on its mobile devices for potential security vulnerabilities, didn't follow commonly accepted secure coding practices, and didn't even respond when warned about the flaws in its devices.

Wyatt, A., Sat Feb 23 2013, B1–2

In 2012, the U.S. government issued a report entitled *A Consumer Privacy Bill of Rights*, whose goal was to establish "a baseline of clear protections for consumers and greater certainty for companies" (Eule, 2013, p. 47). The report argues for consumers' rights to control and transparency while not impeding innovation. A federal Internet policy taskforce was set up in 2013 "to conduct a comprehensive review of the nexus between privacy policy, copyright, global free flow of information, cybersecurity, and innovation in the Internet economy" (National Telecommunications and Information Administration, www. ntia.doc.gov/category/internet-policy-task-force). In the next few years, Congress is expected to consider legislation to protect the privacy of electronic communication. For example, Senator Al Franken of Minnesota introduced the Location Protection Privacy Act 2012, aimed at preventing smartphone apps from tracking location and selling that information to a third party without the smartphone owner's consent (Eule, 2013, p. 47).

5.1 PATIENT AND PROVIDER PRIVACY RISKS ONLINE

To what extent is our patient's privacy at risk of being intruded upon due to the Internet? This is a difficult question to answer precisely, but a reasonable estimate is that the risk is high. Common Sense Media, an organization geared to research and education about digital media use for children and families, has conducted national polls on attitudes towards privacy. Those researchers found that among teenagers, 39% aged 13–17 admitted to having posted content online that they later regretted, and 28% said they had shared personal information online that they would not have shared in person. In 2010, a poll of adults found that 20% had posted personal content that they later regretted. Common Sense Media founder and CEO James Steyer (2012, p. 51) identifies two key problems: first, "self-revealing before self-reflecting," and, second, the inherent conflict in online service providers who stand to gain commercially from aggregating data and the resulting lack of incentive to have effective privacy policies. Steyer, an education professor at Stanford, argues:

> *Taken together, these twin pillars of the broader privacy framework have led to a fundamental change in society's treatment of privacy and the personal lives of millions. This change has occurred virtually overnight, in the span of a few short years, with little public awareness or public leadership and virtually no meaningful public debate" (p. 51).*

In addition to self-revelation without self-reflection, information is obtained about others online in a variety of ways. Facebook stalking, in which online users randomly search others' Facebook pages, is one method. Impersonation and "hacking" occur, in which users pose as the Facebook page owner and change content. Photographs can be "tagged" so that the photo automatically appears on the subject's own Facebook page. (Privacy settings offer a way to prevent tagging, but the default position, as in so many cases of online privacy, is for personal exposure.)

Developing strategies permit increasing interconnectivity in online data. For example, in 2010 Facebook launched "Open Graph." This initiative allowed other websites to put a "Like" button next to pieces of content. By pressing the "Like" button, the content becomes linked to one's Facebook page. *Time* reporter Fletcher uses the example of "Liking" a movie on its website, and then having that being listed under Movies on one's Facebook profile. This strategy allows Facebook to obtain and share more information about the Facebook users and sell it to advertisers for targeting retail advertisements. In 2012, Facebook introduced a similar innovation called "graph search," which allows users to search for others who have "liked" specific topics or locations (Eule, 2013, p. 47).

Another technology called "Timeline" was ostensibly designed to enhance privacy by giving users 7 days to select what they wanted to allow online before it was published. In the words of *New York Times* reporter Jenna Wortham, the technology creates a "scrapbook-like montage" by making "a user's entire history of photos, links and other things shared on Facebook accessible with a single click. This may be the first moment that many of Facebook's 800 million members realize just how many digital bread crumbs they have been leaving on the site – and on the Web in general" (Wortham, 2011, p. 1). Critics of the technology warn that it presents a life's-worth of data in minute detail, providing more fodder for data-miners and snoops.

Concerns about privacy online are such that *Consumer Reports* did a cover story in 2011 projecting that "millions of people jeopardize bank information, medical records, and other sensitive data they store on mobile phones." The article continues:

> *Many active Facebook users take risks than can lead to burglaries, identity theft, and stalking. Fifteen percent had posted their current location or travel plans, 34 percent their full birth date, and 21 percent of those with children at home had posted those children's names and photos. Moreover, roughly one in five [of consumers surveyed] hadn't used Facebook's privacy controls, making them more vulnerable to threats.*
>
> **Consumer Reports, 2011, p. 29**

Moreover, 23% of those surveyed reported being Facebook "friends" with those they didn't know well enough to feel completely comfortable about their own or their family's safety, and an additional 6% said they had a "friend" who made them uncomfortable about security (p. 29).

To what extent is the privacy of health-care professionals at risk of being violated on the Internet? Again, this question is difficult to answer in a precise way. Gorrindo and Groves pointed out in a 2008 commentary that in addition to professional credentials, data about disciplinary actions, malpractice claims, and performance reviews are increasingly available on the Web, as is personal information (Gorrindo & Groves, 2008). A 2010 study by Boston-based physicians found that "personal and professional physician information is widely available on the Internet, and often not under direct control of the individual physician" (Mostaghimi, Crotty & London, 2010, p. 1152). These investigators randomly selected 250 internal medicine physicians registered with the Massachusetts Board of Registration in 2008 and performed "standardized searches" using Google and then analyzed the top 20 search results. In addition, they searched for these physicians on physician-rating sites. They found that 93.6% of the physicians had personal or professional information about them on websites. Of these, 92.8% had professional information and 32.4% had personal information about them online. Female physicians were more likely than male to have online professional information (96.25% v. 91.1%) but the study found no significant gender differences in terms of personal information (p. 1154). The kinds of websites found to hold personal information about physicians were Facebook (10.8%), hobby sites (10.0%), and charitable and political and donation sites (9.6%). Physician-rating sites were found to be the most common sites identified and here the physician information was deemed to be beyond the physicians' control. However, the amount of personal information obtained from these sites was "limited" (Mostaghimi, Crotty & London, 2010, p. 1155).

The study authors pointed out that while most physicians would not discuss with patients in person their political affiliations, or litigation they are involved in, such information is readily available online. Some such information is revealed through online personal disclosure. Some evidence suggests that patients do not welcome in-person self-disclosure, and that it negatively influences how patients experience the quality of care (Beach et al., 2004).

In addition, health-care professionals need to be aware that, increasingly, employers, training programs, insurance providers, health-care institutions, and others are checking online profiles of applicants and prospective employees. Stories abound of hopes being disappointed after negative content about an applicant was discovered online (Cross-Tab 2010; Kahn, 2013; Preston, 2011; Welte [personal communication, May 2012]).

Health-care professionals may be at increased risk for being victim to online harassment and even stalking. "Cyberharassment" typically involves threatening or harassing email messages, blog entries, or websites devoted solely to tormenting an individual. It does not generally include any kind of credible threat. In the United States, 38 states have enacted cyberharassment laws, either by adding language about electronic communication to general harassment statutes, or by creating separate cyberharassment statutes.

For example, a section of one of the Massachusetts General Laws is devoted to Criminal harassment, defined as "willfully and maliciously engag[ing] in a knowing pattern of conduct or series of acts over a period of time directed at a specific person, which seriously alarms that person and would cause a reasonable person to suffer substantial emotional distress." The penalty is up to two-and-a-half years imprisonment, a $1,000 fine, or both. Subsequent language specifies that this conduct includes "acts conducted by... electronic communication device[s] ... including, but not limited to, electronic mail, Internet communications, instant messages or facsimile communications" (accessed from www. malegislature.gov via http://1.usa.gov/x0BZKU).

Cyberharassment of a health-care professional can take the form of directly contacting the professional, for example by email or texting, or of posting undesirable content about them, such as digitally altered photographs of an unprofessional nature. Sexual pictures can be sent to online dating or pornography sites.

"Cyberstalking" is an even more concerning complaint that involves posing a credible threat of harm, often defined as "imminent fear of death or bodily injury" (e.g. see http://1.usa.gov/RYHB0v). Most states in the US now have cyberstalking laws, but not all. If proven, cyberstalking carries more severe sentencing than harassment; for example, in Massachusetts, the sentence is 1–5 years in prison. Unfortunately, because so much information about us is on the

Internet, cyberstalkers can permeate our lives and leave us feeling very vulnerable. Being a victim of cyberstalking can also have a profound impact on how safe we feel in our work, and can generate feelings of anger, fear, and betrayal, all of which we may be at risk of acting out in our work with patients.

Thus far we have discussed privacy intrusion involving information that is inadvertently obtained on the Web or by patients googling us. What about privacy intrusions of patients by their health-care providers? Should health-care professionals google their patients? Chapter 9 discusses the issue of mandated reporting when we learn information about them online, either by performing an online search or inadvertently. In those cases, the issue is what to do with information that may suggest an acute safety issue. But what about when no such safety risks appear to be at hand? Is it wrong to google a patient out of mere curiosity?

Legally, online material is in the public domain; it is not confidential and can be accessed by anyone who chooses to do so. More complicated are the clinical ramifications. What if the discovered content affects how the provider feels about the patient? For example, if it turns out that the patient is very wealthy, or is famous in his area of work, would that inspire undue awe of the patient and lead the quality of care to be different? What if it turns out that the patient and the provider have mutual friends? What if the patient espouses political views that the professional disagrees with? How will the provider handle the discovered information with the patient – keep it secret or disclose it? If the information is kept secret, how will that secret affect the treatment relationship? If disclosed, how will the patient react to the provider having searched online about him or her? What if the provider becomes overly preoccupied with the patient online?

Although their target audience was psychiatrists, Clinton, Silverman, & Brendel (2010) provided a useful framework for health-care professionals to think about "patient targeted-Googling" in the health-care setting. They noted that "Although Internet postings are considered to be in the public domain, the viewing of any information that a patient has not specifically shared in a treatment setting requires careful ethical consideration by clinicians" (p. 104). An online search, they suggest, can be the virtual equivalent of driving by a patient's home or attempting to meet a patient's spouse.

The authors suggest six questions health-care providers should ask themselves before initiating a search about a patient (Box 5.1). First, "Why do I want to conduct this search?" If treaters are motivated by curiosity or frank voyeurism or other interests that place the treater's interest ahead of the patient's, then the treater should not conduct the search. If, on the other hand, the treater honestly feels that searching is in the best interest of the patient, then the treater should move on to

---

BOX 5.1 Six Questions to Ask Yourself Before Googling a Patient

1. Why do I want to conduct this search?
2. Would my search advance or compromise the treatment?
3. Should I obtain informed consent from the patient prior to searching?
4. Should I share the results of the search with the patient?
5. Should I document the findings of the search in the medical record?
6. How do I monitor my motivations and the ongoing risk–benefit profile of searching?

Clinton, B. K., Silverman, B. D., & Brendel, D. H. (2010). Patient-targeted Googling: The ethics of searching online for patient information. Harvard Review of Psychiatry, 18, 103–112.

---

question 2: "Would my search advance or compromise the treatment?" An important aspect of this question is whether the information needs to be obtained online, or whether it can more prudently be obtained via other sources, including interviewing the patient. In some cases, for example, when struggling to locate a relative of an elderly patient who has become delirious, an online search may be warranted. The third question is whether informed consent needs to be obtained prior to searching. This question gets us back to the definition of privacy quoted by Buckovich, Rippen, & Rozen (1999, p. 123): "freedom from intrusion or observation into one's private affairs, [and] the right to maintain control over certain personal information." Informed consent is a means of giving the patient control over their personal information, and mitigating any negative feelings the patient may experience (hurt, anger, betrayal) if a search is not initially disclosed but subsequently discovered.

Question 4 is: "Should I share the results of the search with the patient?" This is another question whose answer rests in the details of the specific doctor–patient relationship and the characteristics of each person, especially the patient. When in doubt, consultation is advised.

What about documenting the findings from the search in the medical record? (see Question 5). Documentation raises a further level of complication because, of course, patients have access to their medical records, which nowadays includes online access. If the information relates to medical decision-making, it probably should be documented. If it is compromising to the patient or casts him or her in a negative light, (e.g. elicit drug use), the information should probably be discussed with the patient before being documented. Again, legal, ethical, and clinical consultation may be warranted.

Finally, Clinton et al. suggest question 6: How do I monitor my motivations and ongoing risk–benefit profile of searching going forward? This question requires honest introspection on the part of the provider. When providers are hurried, stressed, in emotionally depleted states, or otherwise vulnerable, they may be more likely to deceive themselves about their motivations and, as a result, get themselves into trouble. Like much online activity, the positive reinforcement of obtaining intimate information about a patient can result in Internet addiction kinds of behaviors. Any provider who has become immersed in online searches of patients or one particular patient should seek a mental health consultation.

Sometimes, patients are eager to show us their online activity. In such a case, it may be appropriate to look online with the patient as long as patient privacy is not compromised by content that is on the professional's desk or visible on the computer (Gabbard et al, 2012, p. 66).

5.2 VIGNETTES

Let us now turn to specific case examples to see how these privacy concerns can play out in clinical practice and think through how to approach potential problems.

Vignette 5.1

A male pediatrician notes that a long-time patient, a male adolescent, has uncharacteristically canceled two recent appointments. The pediatrician calls the patient to ask if there are any problems, and the patient reluctantly admits that he had googled the physician and found photos of him participating in a recent Gay Pride parade. The patient had been unaware that his physician was gay and felt that he should have been told about his doctor's sexual orientation.

Adapted from DeJong, et al, 2011, Vignette #9

The first step when confronted with unexpected information is not to become defensive. Defensiveness shuts communication down and elevates feelings so that rational discussion is not possible. We want to keep the conversation open in order to better understand why the patient looked for the information, what impact the information had on the patient, and how it affected the patient's view of the professional. For example, in the vignette above, the young adolescent may be struggling with his own sexual identity. Perhaps he started to feel attracted to his physician. Or perhaps he experienced this attraction, or his conflicted feelings, as homophobia. Or perhaps he was just playing around on his computer and got the idea in his head of googling people in his life. The pediatrician, recognizing the no-show behavior as atypical for this patient, reaches out.

One can easily imagine the pediatrician feeling defensive. If he is not "out" in his professional community, discovering that his sexual orientation is broadcast on the Internet might feel like a personal violation. He may feel angry that his personal life is being exposed, and that this exposure is coming between him and his young patient. If anger gets the best of him, the pediatrician might respond on the telephone by saying he is sorry the patient feels that way and he would be happy to refer him to a heterosexual pediatrician. But such action is likely not in the best interests of the patient.

In fact, the next best step will probably be for the pediatrician to invite the patient in to discuss what he has learned and how he feels about it. In that way, the pediatrician has the opportunity to maintain a professional identity and try to preserve the treatment alliance. The conversation could actually deepen the doctor–patient relationship by providing an opportunity for the patient to discuss his own conflicted feelings about sexuality.

Of course, the patient's and the professional's experience of discovered information will vary according to the type of information. If a patient learns that a physician belongs to one political party and the patient belongs to another, the patient may feel that these political views represent such a great obstacle to an ongoing relationship that a change of practitioner is necessary. Interestingly, for healthcare professionals, our professionalism mandate is to show cross-cultural sensitivity, to care for the person who is our patient, and not allow our own biases to get in the way. Successfully practicing in this way can become increasingly challenging as we may inadvertently learn more and more about our patients.

Vignette 5.2

A nurse practitioner has just had her third visit with a patient. About this time, she is "friended" on Facebook by an old high school classmate. However, the communications from the "classmate" do not appear to be genuine; in fact, this person appears to be an imposter. The nurse practitioner is able to ascertain from information on the imposter's Facebook page that the "friend" is actually the patient (who had located the nurse practitioner's high school yearbook online).

Adapted from DeJong et al., 2011, Vignette #1

This is an example of online impersonation. One of the great difficulties of online communication is that it is often impossible to verify who is at the other end of a textual posting. Fortunately, the nurse practitioner in this case was observant and recognized inconsistencies on the Facebook exchange that alerted her to the impersonation. What to do now? Much will depend on the personality and emotional stability of the patient. Given the need for a detailed understanding of this patient in order to know how best to proceed, clinical and legal consultations are warranted. Ideally, the nurse practitioner will be able to gently confront the patient about the impersonation, empathically explore the motivations behind it, and come to agreement about reasonable privacy boundaries for patient and practitioner alike.

When patients are less emotionally stable or even personality-disordered, the situation can be much more difficult, as in the following vignette.

Vignette 5.3

A psychotherapist is seeing a patient in psychotherapy for treatment of ongoing depression and interpersonal difficulties consistent with borderline personality disorder. The patient becomes deeply connected to her therapist, and relies on him heavily for emotional wellbeing. However, in one session the therapist and patient disagree about how best to manage a personal situation in the patient's life. The patient experiences a lack of empathy from her treater, and begins to feel angry with him. The degree of the patient's rage is largely unconscious to the patient, who goes online to learn personal information about the therapist who has, in her mind, betrayed her.

Soon, the therapist is receiving threatening emails and Facebook postings from the patient detailing personal information about the therapist's life. Then, the therapist's colleagues begin to receive messages on their Facebook pages from the patient, castigating the therapist and explicitly threatening anyone who associates with him.

This vignette is an example of cyberstalking, and is obviously a gross violation of the health-care provider's privacy and a highly aggressive act. The threats are to be taken seriously, for even experienced mental health professionals cannot predict how patients are going to behave. See Recommendation 8 below for advice on how to manage cyberharassment and cyberstalking.

Vignette 5.4

A director of training for surgery during recruitment season is very interested in a particular candidate's resume, which lists some intriguing research papers. In order to locate one of the papers, the training director googles the candidate's name and finds that she has been regularly involved with paraphilic noncriminal sexual activities (S&M) and there are some provocative photos of her available online.

Adapted from DeJong et al., 2011, Vignette #10

Do training programs and employers that routinely perform online searches of applicants as part of the screening process have an obligation to inform the applicants ahead of time? Standards are changing around these issues, but media reports and the Cross-Tab survey (p. 69) suggest such online screenings of applicants are increasingly commonplace. Health-care professionals would be wise to err on the side of caution and not disclose any kind of potentially compromising information about themselves online. If a search is conducted that has an impact on the trainee or the prospective employee, the decision whether to disclose the findings to that person is a complex one and may again depend on specific details of the case.

Vignette 5.5

A medical trainee in a rural residency has a large number of Facebook "friends" that include non-medical professionals, colleagues in training, and supervising physicians. In a conversation with a training colleague, the trainee learns that two of her friends, this colleague and a supervisor, are in a doctor–patient relationship.

Adapted from DeJong et al, 2011, Vignette #30

This vignette addresses the issue of developing online relationships across health-care hierarchies and, inadvertently, within a treatment frame. In this case, a medical supervisor and a trainee are Facebook "friends of friends." Moreover, they are in a treatment relationship. Is this inherently wrong? Probably not. However, a communication doorway is now open: If the training colleague reveals anything about her treatment or her treater without knowing that the supervisor is also a "friend on the page," the trainee may feel that her privacy has not been protected. Does the owner of the site have a duty to "protect" her friend and let her know that the supervisor is also a Facebook "friend"? The answer to that question may lie in the specific details of the case, but should certainly be considered. Hierarchies also tend to generate some sense of hierarchical privacy: In general, trainees do not know the intimate details of their supervisors' lives and vice versa. Cutting across peer groups in this fashion starts to blur privacy boundaries, although, as we have discussed, "millennials" tend to respect hierarchies less than baby-boomers. In addition, one might wonder what would happen if other trainees learn that some trainees are "friends" with the supervisor but not others. The training situation itself may no longer be viewed as a level playing field, but rather one in which teachers play favorites.

5.3 GENERAL RECOMMENDATIONS

Specific recommendations listed by technology are discussed in Chapter 11. Some general principles to protect physician and patient privacy are reviewed here:

1. Think before clicking to avoid revealing personal content before reflecting on potential repercussions of the disclosure, including clinical and professional. Encourage your colleagues and patients to do the same.
2. Be familiar with developing guidelines around disclosure. A growing number of health-care organizations, professional societies, malpractice insurers, and licensing boards are setting restrictions on what is acceptable content for health-care professionals to post online.
3. Perform online audits of content about yourself. By searching for your own name online, you will find what your patients are finding, and have an opportunity to change it before they see it. How to deal with unwanted content is discussed in Chapter 12.
4. Generate positive content about yourself online. A professional website with accurate, useful health information will rise to the top of the search list the more it is accessed, and less desirable content will move down the search list.
5. Access legal, ethical and clinical consultation if needed, and consider the services of a professional online privacy firm (see Chapter 11).
6. In general, health-care professionals should only conduct online searches about patients when, after careful thought, they feel they are driven by motivation to serve the patient (as opposed to curiosity or voyeurism), and are clear whether consent is needed and what they will do with the information obtained.
7. Expect that patients will google you and prepare ahead of time how you will respond to various kinds of information they may reveal about you. Consider asking patients whether they have googled you in the event that the treatment relationship has changed.
8. What should health-care professionals do if they fall victim to cyberharassment or cyberstalking? Security expert Mary Kay Hoal (Hoal, 2012) offers five approaches. First, recognize

cyberharassment when you see it. Do not try to engage with the person. Harassers, like bullies, often feed off their victim's pain, and responding can make matters worse. Second, make a copy of the message, photo or video. Hoal advises both a URL and a screenshot of the webpage. For a website, contact the website operators requesting they take the content down. Persistence may be key to success. File a report with your local police department. If necessary file a complaint with the Internet Crime Complaint Center (IC3). The IC3 is a partnership between the FBI, the National White Collar Crime Center, and the Bureau of Justice Assistance. They work together on serious cases of online criminal complaints in the USA. In addition, obtain clinical and, if necessary, psychotherapeutic consultation to think through the inevitable impact of such a frightening experience on your work as a practitioner and the potential need for ongoing psychological support.

9. Increasingly, efforts are underway to prevent anonymous postings. Practitioners should be aware of the regulations around anonymous postings in their own health-care websites and jurisdictions.

CONCLUSION

Privacy is distinct from confidentiality in that it pertains not just to information but to the overall right of a person to be free of unwanted intrusions. In health care, laws protect the privacy and confidentiality of patients and information derived from their care. General privacy laws protect privacy rights of individuals, but being emailed or "friended" by a patient has not, at the time of writing, been viewed as a privacy violation; health-care providers have little protection from unwanted online intrusions. In general, strong feelings are elicited when individuals perceive their privacy to have been violated, including anger and betrayal. For this reason, professionals would do well to respect the privacy of their patients and not perform online searches about them unless they are convinced that it is the only way to obtain necessary information to advance the patient's care. In such a case, they should consider obtaining patient consent. Any information that is learned inadvertently may need to be discussed explicitly with the patient in terms of its impact on the treatment relationship.

In contrast, professionals should expect that patients will be searching online about them and prepare for the impact of such information on the treatment relationship, regardless of whether the patient discloses or keeps secret what has been learned. Practitioners should make reasonable efforts to protect their own privacy, including not posting online any content they would not wish patients to know.

Such a double standard may frustrate health-care professionals. If Im an open book to my patients, why can't they be an open book to me? Or, if I work so hard to protect the privacy of my patients, why can't they reciprocate? The answer lies again in the fiduciary nature of the professional relationship we hold with our patients. By definition, they are putting trust in health-care professionals in a relationship where they are the vulnerable party. One important exception to patients' rightful ability to learn about us online is "cyberharassment" and "cyberstalking," in which providers and even their loved ones are threatened by their patients online. Cyberstalking requires involvement of law enforcement and careful clinical and psychological consultation.

REFERENCES

Appelbaum, P. S., & Gutheil, T. G. (2007). *Clinical handbook of psychiatry and the law*. Philadelphia, PA: Wolters Kluwer/Lippincott Williams & Wilkins.

Beach, M. C., Roter, D., Rubin, H., Frankel, R., Levinson, W., & Ford, D. E. (2004). Is physician self-disclosure related to patient evaluation of office visits? *Journal of General Internal Medicine*, *19*, 905–910.

Buckovich, S. A., Rippen, H. E., & Rozen, M. J. (1999). Driving toward guiding principles: A goal for privacy, confidentiality, and security of health information. *Journal of the American Medical Informatics Association*, *6*, 122–133. http://dx.doi.org/10.1135/jamia.1999.0060122.

Clinton, B. K., Silverman, B. C., & Brendel, D. H. (2010). Patient-targeted googling: The ethics of searching online for patient information. *Harvard Review of Psychiatry*, *18*, 103–112.

Consumer Reports, (2011). Online exposure – Social networks, mobile phones, and scams can threaten your security. *Consumer Reports*, *76*(6), 29–33.

Cross-Tab, (2010). Online reputation in a connected world. Retrieved from <www.slideshare.net> via <http://slidesha.re/cp2wV0>.

DeJong, S. et al. (2011). Curriculum on professionalism and the Internet in psychiatry. Retrieved from <www.aadprt.org> via <http://bit.ly/Yh1JRq>.

Egan, J. (2010). *A Visit from the Goon Squad*. New York, NY: Anchor Books.

Eule, B. (2013). Can I get some privacy? *Stanford Magazine*, March/April, 45–49.

Fienberg, S. E. (2006). Privacy and confidentiality in an e-commerce world: Data mining, data warehousing, matching and disclosure limitation. *Statistical Science*, *21*(2), 143–154. http://dx.doi.org/10.1214/088342306000000240.

Fletcher, D. (2010). Facebook: Friends without borders. *Time*, *175*(21), 33–38.

Fox, M. (2013). Alan F. Westin, who transformed privacy debate before the web era, dies at 83. *The New York Times,* February 23, A17.

Gabbard, G. O., Roberts, L. W., Crisp-Han, H., Ball, V., Hobday, G., & Rachal, F (2012). *Professionalism in Psychiatry*. Washington, DC: American Psychiatric Press.

Gorrindo, T., & Groves, J. E. (2008). Web-searching for information about physicians. *Journal of the American Medical Association*, *300*(2), 213–215. http://dx.doi.org/doi:10.1001/jama.2008.44.

Gymrek, M., McGuire, A. L., Golan, D., Halperin, E., & Erlich, Y. (2013). Identifying personal genomes by surname inference. *Science*, *339*, 321–324. http://dx.doi.org/doi:10.1126/science.1229566.

Harris, J. A., Levy, A. R., & Teschke, K. E. (2008). Personal privacy and public health: Potential impacts of privacy legislation on human research in Canada. *Canadian Journal of Public Health*, *99*(4), 293–296.

Hoal, M.K. (2012). Five ways to handle and prevent cyber-harassment. <Retrieved from abcnews.go.com>.

Johnson, C.V. (2013). Using simple tools, scientists show privacy of research participants is at risk. *The Boston Globe*, January 17, p. 1.

Kahn, J.P. (2013). E-trails of trouble – young job-hunters fix online selves. *The Boston Globe*, February 14, A1, A8.

Kass, N. E., et al. (2004). Medical privacy and the disclosure of personal medical information: The beliefs and experiences of those with genetic and other clinical conditions. *American Journal of Medical Genetics*, *128A*, 261–270.

Malamud Smith, J. (2003). *Privacy Matters: In Defense of the Personal Life*. Emeryville, CA: Seal Press.

Mostaghimi, A., Crotty, B. H., & Landon, B. E. (2010). The availability and nature of physician information on the internet. *Journal of General Internal Medicine*, *25*(11), 1152–1156. http://dx.doi.org/10.1007/s11606-010-1425-7.

Nelson, K. (2011). Confidentiality vs privacy. <Inpropriapersona.com>. Retrieved from <http://inpropriapersona.com/confidentiality-vs-privacy/>.

Partners Healthcare, undated. Confidentiality vs privacy and how they relate to human subjects protections. Retrieved from <http://www.healthcare.partners.org/phsirb/confidentiality_privacy.htm>.

Perritt, H. H. (n.d.). Regulatory models for protecting privacy on the internet. In National Telecommunications and information administration, models for self-regulation. Retrieved from <http://www.ntia.doc.gov/page/chapter-3-models-self-regulation>.

Preston, J. (2011). Social media history becomes a new job hurdle. *The New York Times,* July 20.

Steyer, J. P. (2012). *Talking Back to Facebook – the common sense guide to raising kids in the digital age*. New York: Scribner.

Westin, A. F. (1968). *Privacy and Freedom*. New York: Atheneum.

Wortham, J., (2011). Your life on Facebook, in total recall. *The New York Times*, December 15. Retrieved from <www.nytimes.com> via <http://nyti.ms/XJbkjX>.

Chapter | Six

Libel

Most democratic countries protect their citizens' right to free speech. In the United States, it is protected in the Constitution under the First Amendment. As a result, patients are welcome to talk online and in digital media about their medical providers. Tweeting, texting, blogging, and posting on social media sites like Tumblr and Facebook all provide opportunities for patients to describe their experience in treatment.

Increasingly, online rating sites such as healthgrades.com and ratemds.com, as well as the more generic rating sites like Angie's list, provide an opportunity for systematic ranking and evaluation of health-care professionals. In a study of information about physicians on the Internet, quality-rating sites were the most common way in which information about physicians was available on the Internet. Over 70% of physicians surveyed in this study were on Healthgrades, 13.2% on RateMD, and 38.4% on Wellness (Mostaghimi, Crotty & Landon, 2010, p. 1155).

At the same time, the law protects individuals from damaging falsehoods. Such protection is particularly true for private citizens, as opposed to public figures who are deemed to be putting themselves voluntarily in the public eye. In American law, "defamation" is the term for "Any intentional false communication, either written or spoken, that harms a person's reputation; decreases the respect, regard, or confidence in which a person is held; or induces disparaging, hostile, or disagreeable opinions or feelings against a person" (http://legal-dictionary.thefreedictionary.com/defamation). Plaintiffs can bring defamation complaints against individuals under either criminal or civil law. Slander is the legal term for oral defamation – untrue spoken comments that are shown to harm the

S. deJong: Blogs and Tweets, Texting and Friending.
DOI: http://dx.doi.org/10.1016/B978-0-12-408128-4.00006-0
© 2014 S. DeJong. Published by Elsevier Inc. All rights reserved.

individual about whom the remarks are made. Libel is the written form of defamation, which includes broadcast or online content. The law distinguishes inadvertent from malicious communication of untrue content; damages awarded are typically higher when malice has been shown. Government organizations and public records are typically immune from libel, with some exceptions.

Another important distinction in defamation is that the statement must be made as fact rather than opinion. Thus, a comment that "The nurse who assisted in the birth of my baby was the worst nurse I've ever had" is an opinion to which the commenter is entitled. However, a comment like "That incompetent doctor is practicing without a license" states as fact that the physician is an unlicensed provider which, if true, would mean that the physician was breaking the law and, if untrue, might constitute defamation.

Finally, successful defamation lawsuits require demonstration of harm. Thus, in the example above of the allegedly unlicensed physician, it would need to be proved that the individual's false allegation resulted in damage to the physician's reputation and good name. Examples of harm might be a decrease in the number of referrals to one's practice; being asked to step down from professional organizations; being attacked generally in the media; and so on. Distinguishing harmful, factual statements from harmless opinion can be difficult. Let us look at some examples.

6.1 VIGNETTES

Vignette 6.1

A nurse on a surgical service learns from a medical student that comments about her have been posted on the Facebook page of a recently discharged patient. The medical student had become a "friend" on Facebook with the patient, and seen the comments, which refer to the nurse as "Nurse Cratchett" and criticize her "bitchy" manner and down-to-business approach to patient care. When the medical student shows the postings to the nurse, the latter is offended, particularly because she views herself as highly professional and has received awards from her hospital for her clinical care. She wants to pursue legal action.

In this case, the patient is expressing an opinion about the nurse. Like many opinions, this one may not be well thought out or based on solid evidence. In fact, the opinion may say more about the patient than it does about the nurse: Perhaps the patient was feeling vulnerable and in particular need of a maternal caring style; perhaps the patient had had bad experiences in life with nurses; or perhaps the patient was attracted to the nurse and tried to reach out to her but felt no response. The nurse may well never know. But regardless of the patient's conscious or unconscious motives for posting the opinion about the nurse, it remains an opinion – not a fact – and any legal action is probably unwarranted and unrealistic.

This second example is perhaps less clear cut.

Vignette 6.2

An early-career psychiatrist discovers that someone has submitted a negative review of him on an online physician-rating site. The writer alleges that the psychiatrist "occasionally violated my civil rights." The psychiatrist is concerned about the potential impact to his reputation as he begins practice if this review is available on the website. He suspects the writer is a former patient with chronic mental illness who presented regularly to the emergency room during his training and had occasionally to be psychiatrically committed to the inpatient unit against his will. The psychiatrist considers whether to submit positive reviews under various pseudonyms, pretending that they are written by real patients, to create a more favorable impression of the psychiatrist on the website.

DeJong et al., 2011, Vignette #15

In this case, the specific allegation that the psychiatrist violated the patient's civil rights is made as a statement of fact. This example also points to the difficulty of online ratings that do not necessarily require people either to identify themselves or to offer full disclosure in terms of their relationship to the particular health-care provider. In this case, an online audience might view the rater and the review differently if the rater made it more explicit that he is chronically mentally ill. A wise consumer of online information might do well to take all such posted information with a grain of salt. Nonetheless, the allegation of civil rights violations is starting to move from opinion to factual statement.

What is less clear from the vignette is what potential harm the presumably false allegation might have on the young psychiatrist. For a defamation case to go forward, the psychiatrist would need to be able to demonstrate that this posting by a single individual has had a negative impact on his reputation or professional standing. Such a case would seem difficult to make. However, to take matters into his own hands by posing as other patients and writing more favorable reviews is hardly a favorable alternative. Two wrongs, in this case, do not make a right: Falsifying one's identity online is unethical.

In the following example, the risk of harm, in this case to an endocrinologist, would appear to be greater.

Vignette 6.3

An endocrinologist is informed by a current patient that a former patient (whom the current patient knows from a group for people with diabetes) has been systematically logging on to blogs, websites, and chat rooms for patients with diabetes and saying negative things that are untrue about the endocrinologist. The physician goes online to verify these allegations and finds a number of sites on which the patient has not only named her but also alleged that she is both "incompetent" and "practicing without a license." The patient reports that his health declined under the care of the endocrinologist, and urges others not to see them.

Adapted from DeJong et al., 2011, Vignette #16

This vignette exemplifies a patient systematically seeking to defame the reputation of a health-care professional. Given the prevalence of the postings and the serious nature of the allegations, the potential harm to the endocrinologist's reputation would seem significant. If the allegations are false, they could constitute libel.

6.2 GENERAL RECOMMENDATIONS REGARDING LIBEL ONLINE

What can health-care professionals do to protect themselves against defamatory online postings? False information that is stated as fact can and should be changed. For example, a dentist who was reported on a state government website as having had disciplinary action taken against him for illegal conduct should request a correction. Ensuring that professional websites such as medical boards display correct information about us is an important responsibility.

If negative content does not cause frank harm but does bruise narcissistic feelings, peer or professional support should be sought to prevent acting-out behaviors. All of us have feelings in the face of negative feedback or criticism. Health-care professionals can easily become angry, defensive or hostile in the face of negative content on rating sites. If the defamatory comments are widespread or serious enough that the professional believes harm has been done, then legal consultation should be pursued. Finally, "reputation-defending" services are now available. "Reputation.com," "reputationadvocate.com," and "internetreputation.com" are all examples of such companies that advertise with slogans such as, "People don't ask for character references anymore, they ask Google" (http://www.reputation.com/myreputation). For thousands of dollars a year, these companies work on hiding negative online content about their clients. However, as even they admit, for the most part such negative content cannot be deleted.

Of course, health-care professionals themselves can also use strategies to affect the order in which content about them presents on an online search. Creating positive content that will generate multiple "hits," such as a professional website, a well-written blog, or articles available online through open-access, are examples of such an approach. Other methods are discussed in Chapter 11.

Increasingly, online sources are encouraging accountability by limiting anonymous postings. For example, in New York State, legislation filed in Albany, the Internet Protection Act, would require sites to remove anonymous postings unless the poster agrees to attach his or her name to the post (Huffington Post, 2012). Such efforts towards more transparency and accountability may decrease the number of false and damaging statements about health-care professionals online.

CONCLUSION

Libel is the term for false, harmful, written (including digitally) statements about an individual. Health-care professionals who find false content about themselves on professional websites such as state licensing boards should request that the information be corrected. However, a whole host of other websites and media on the Internet provide a vast opportunity for the expression of feelings and opinions about health-care providers. Opinion alone does not constitute libel, and negative opinions about one's professional performance or identity are best ignored and handled with equanimity. However, statements of "fact" which are untrue and risk providing significant harm to the provider merit legal consultation. Performing regular online inventories to learn what is being said about us online is vital. More specific recommendations will be discussed in Chapter 11.

REFERENCES

DeJong, S. et al. (2011). Curriculum on professionalism and the Internet in psychiatry. Retrieved from <www.aadprt.org> via <http://bit.ly/Yh1JRq>.

Huffington Post. (2012). Internet Protection Act would eliminate anonymous online comments in New York. Retrieved from <www.huffingtonpost.com> via <http://huff.to/ZwueLq>.

Mostaghimi, A., Crotty, B. H., & Landon, B. E. (2010). The availability and nature of physician information on the internet. *Journal of General Internal Medicine*, *25*(11), 1152–1156. http://dx.doi.org/doi:10.1007/s11606-010-1425-7.

Chapter Seven

Conflicts of Interest

Appropriate handling of actual and potential conflicts of interest is a key professionalism skill. As with many professionalism and ethical issues, the first step is recognizing when conflict of interest may be playing a role in any given situation. Once recognized, a conflict of interest can be worked through, although often not completely resolved, in a professional manner. The American Academy of Child and Adolescent Psychiatry (www.aacap.org) usefully discusses conflict of interest in terms of the "four A-s":

- Awareness of obligation to their patients and to maintain integrity
- Assessment of potential conflicts of interest in their practice
- Acknowledgment of how these conflicts may affect decision-making
- Action by reporting and managing potential conflicts of interest when dealing with patients and colleagues.

7.1 WHAT IS A CONFLICT OF INTEREST?

In 2009, the Institute of Medicine (IOM) issued a report entitled *Conflict of Interest in Medical Research, Education and Practice* in which the authors define conflict of interest as "a set of circumstances that creates a risk that professional judgment or actions regarding a primary interest will be unduly influenced by a secondary influence." For most health-care professionals, our primary interest as defined by the IOM is "promoting and protecting … the welfare of patients" (IOM, 2009, p. 25). However, health-care professionals often wear many hats and play a number of different roles in the course of their work. Thus, many of us have competing primary interests when we work not only as practitioners but also as researchers, consultants, administrators, educators, writers, board members, forensic experts, and so on.

S. deJong: Blogs and Tweets, Texting and Friending.
DOI: http://dx.doi.org/10.1016/B978-0-12-408128-4.00007-2
© 2014 S. DeJong. Published by Elsevier Inc. All rights reserved.

Let us look at an illustration. An academic physician may be primarily a researcher, but also see patients, teach medical students, and sit on a number of organizational boards. Sometimes these roles can come into conflict; if the physician is running a research study on a medication, and he has a patient whom he believes would benefit from the medication, that physician may try to recruit the patient into the study. Although his conscious intent may be to help the patient, he also stands to benefit by recruiting another subject into his study; thus, a conflict of interest arises. This situation demonstrates why in research studies physicians may be prohibited from recruiting their own patients, lest coercion play a role.

All of us also have what the IOM calls "secondary interests," i.e. personal interests which benefit us but not necessarily our patients. These include financial benefit, the wish for professional advancement, and professional standing in our field. These secondary interests are human and not in and of themselves unethical. However, they too can consciously and unconsciously play a role in how we behave in our primary role of taking care of patients and in our more secondary roles.

To what extent health-care professionals should allow secondary interests to come into play in their work has been a historic debate. The Scottish philosopher-physician John Gregory, who wrote the first modern, professional medical ethics guide in the English language (*Lectures on the Duties and Qualifications of a Physician*, 1772), argued that physicians' service should not be determined by financial reward but by the virtue of self-sacrifice. Even today, health-care reform advocates like physician Arnold Relman argue that confounding the profession of medicine with business interests through the recent development of private, non-investor-owned insurance plans and health-care facilities inevitably raised conflicts of interest:

*Physicians became associated with them as investors,
owners, partners, or employees, thus creating financial
conflicts of interest that were unprecedented in number
and variety. Even when they deliberately avoided such
association and confined their sources of income to the care
of patients, physicians increasingly thought of themselves
as private business people, competing with their colleagues
for a share of the patient market. With the growth of medical
technology and the ever-increasing specialization and
subspecialization of medical and surgical practice, the
financial rewards of entrepreneurial behavior continue to
grow ... Medicine never in its history totally rejected the
seductions of financial gain, but until fairly recently most*

young physicians entered their profession with the primary
intention to be of service to their patients … [F]inancial
ambition did not trump professional ethics, as it increasingly
seems to do now.

Relman, 2007, p. 376

Others have argued that such concerns are exaggerated (IOM, 2009).

7.2 MANAGING CONFLICTS OF INTEREST

Like so many ethical quandaries, the dilemmas involved in conflict of interest rarely have a single answer. Resolving them often involves identifying and attempting to balance the various competing interests. For example, in determining whether a financial relationship constitutes a conflict of interest, and, if so, how important the conflict is and how it should be managed, the IOM recommends considering the following: How important is the secondary interest or relationship for furthering primary medical values? What is the likelihood and seriousness of possible harm to those primary values? Are measures to reduce the likelihood or severity of harm available? (IOM, 2009, p. 56). Sometimes more information in the form of research or consultation is needed to answer these questions.

Several methods to prevent and address conflicts of interest can be mobilized once the conflicts have been identified (Gabbard et al., 2012). The growing number of institutional and organizational conflict of interest policies is an effort to do just that. Although difficult to do consistently, in some cases assuming multiple roles can be avoided. For example, one might decline to write a review of a book written by a friend. Increasingly, medical professionals are required to disclose potential conflicts of interest so that others can assess to what extent secondary interests may be affecting behavior in the primary area of work. Limits may need to be set by institutions and oversight bodies to minimize undue interests. For example, medical clinics may develop a policy prohibiting all "free" products donated by pharmaceutical companies. Providing ongoing information and education may also be a useful strategy to heighten awareness and minimize negative consequences around real and perceived conflicts of interest. Of course, all policies will need to be revised and monitored appropriately. By taking these measures, institutions and, indeed, the whole health-care profession can preserve public trust and promote a "culture of accountability that sustains professional norms and promotes public confidence in professional judgments" (IOM, 2009, p. 29). Our failure to monitor ourselves runs the risk of increasing pressure for external regulation (p. 30).

7.3 CONFLICTS OF INTEREST, SOCIAL MEDIA AND THE INTERNET

How does this background on conflict of interest relate to digital technology and the Internet? As with so many professionalism concerns in the digital age, it is not so much that new technologies raise brand new issues as that the opportunity for potential breaches is broader and their potential impact more rapid, more widespread, and more permanent. On the bright side, because various roles that we play may be made public and easily accessible by the Internet, the opportunity for greater transparency may exist. The potential issues may be most usefully discussed through specific examples.

7.3.1 Vignettes

Blogging is an online activity many health-care professionals engage in, and the number of professional websites has been steadily increasing. Technorati, a Web-tracking service, estimated that in 2007 about 70 million blogs were online and about 120,000 more were being created each day. Let us look at a blogging vignette.

> **Vignette 7.1**
>
> *A physician who has expertise in substance abuse treatment writes a blog about substance abuse and dependence disorders and their treatment. The blog includes up-to-date information about substances and their effects on the brain and the body, and current research in the field. The physician's name and contact information are clearly stated at the top of the blog. The physician also snail-mails all members of the local medical society a postcard advertising the blog, describing it as one of the "top-rated medical blogs in the country" and boasts about "hundreds of blog posts and subscribers," both of which are true statements. At the bottom of the postcard in fine print is a statement regarding substance abuse services being available on a fee-for-service basis.*
>
> Here, the blog itself may contain useful information for patients. The author of the information is identified – it is not an anonymous blog; thus, "consumers," i.e. potential patients, are free to look up the credentials of the practitioner. Nonetheless, it is the kind of content to which Dr. Relman (cited above) might object; it appears to be an "infomercial" – informational content that functions to advertise a private practice which treats patients outside of insurance reimbursement. This activity is legal and widely used. However, it does raise the potential issue of conflict of interest. Which hat does this physician wear in writing his blog – the clinician hat which carries with it the primary interest in the care of patients, or the small-business-owner hat which necessitates a primary interest in making a profit? How do his dual and presumably sometimes competing interests play out in the clinical setting?

This tension between a doctor's own interest and the interest of the patient or consumer may also come into play in online endorsements. In a study of 271 medical blogs, 11.4% of the blogs studied contained promotions of health-care products (Lagu, Kaufman, Asch & Armstrong, 2008). Consider the following hypothetical example:

Vignette 7.2

A physician develops a cell phone application that enables graphing and transmission of the smartphone user's vital signs. The physician then goes to the online stores which market the application and writes glowing reviews. The physician also distributes brochures about the product, and how to purchase it, in the waiting room of his private office and on his professional website.

In this case, the physician has a clear conflict of interest: He is endorsing a product whose sale he stands to benefit from directly. Online anonymous reviews (such as those found on Amazon and Yelp) make it easy for us all to engage in these potential conflicts. In general, endorsing one's own work (be it medical products, written articles or books) without disclosure of the potential conflict would be considered unethical.

There is an additional professionalism concern in this vignette: As discussed above, many Institutional Review Boards express concern when health-care professionals who are also research investigators attempt to recruit their own patients into their research studies. Their reasoning is concern about coercion given the special relationship between professional and patient and the frequent power differential. Will the patients feel comfortable saying no to their treater, or will they say yes to please the treater, aspiring to win favored status? When physicians advertise their own products directly to their patients, as above, a similar concern is raised. More vulnerable patients, especially, may have a need to ingratiate themselves to their health-care provider by buying the product. Some may expect a *quid pro quo* – if I do this for you, I expect you to do something for me. Some may harbor resentment about being the target of the provider's advertising and the resentment may get explicitly expressed or implicitly reflected in the patient's behavior toward the health-care provider.

Such situations are not limited to endorsements of the health-care professional's own products. Endorsing medications if one owns stock in the pharmaceutical company that produces it, endorsing systems of care such as specific hospitals if one has a professional relationship with it, or endorsing a professional organization if one stands to gain by others joining it – are all examples of potential conflicts of interest that need to be managed, typically by explicit disclosure of the conflict. Here is an example:

Vignette 7.3

On her professional blog, a physician's assistant (PA) extols the virtues of a new cholesterol-lowering medication in treating patients with high cholesterol. She mentions several patients whose cholesterol levels have been significantly lowered after they started the medication. The PA does not disclose that having seen these clinical results, she purchased stock in the manufacturer of the medication.

Here, the PA is expressing a professional opinion based on clinical experience without disclosing the obvious potential conflict that she stands to gain financially from the sale of the medication. The PA could have chosen to share the results of clinical studies on her blog, rather than the weaker scientific evidence of anecdotal experience. Nonetheless, she would need to disclose her ownership of the stock in order to allow the reader/consumer to have the necessary information to consider whether her assessment of the product might be biased by her financial interest.

Not all endorsement conflicts of interest stem from self-interest: In some cases, health-care professionals may want to endorse not-for-profit activities. Consider this vignette:

Vignette 7.4

A physician practices in a public-sector clinic and is on the board of a local homeless shelter and food pantry located in the same neighborhood as the clinic. In preparation for an annual fundraiser for the shelter, the physician writes on his blog about the importance of the shelter to the community. He also participates in an email campaign soliciting donations from friends and neighbors.

Here, the physician's efforts would seem to be in the interests of the shelter rather than himself. Nonetheless, he seems to hold two different roles in the community, as clinician and as board member of the shelter. The physician may not perceive any potential conflict in these roles, but it may be prudent for him to disclose his clinic role in his online fundraising activities so that participants in the fundraiser have the necessary knowledge to make that determination.

These kinds of seemingly altruistic endeavors might fall into the category of the health-care professional's own personal values and beliefs, which are often inextricably linked to who the professional is as a person. Thus, the gay pediatrician whose photograph at the Gay Pride parade was seen online by an adolescent patient unwittingly revealed not only his apparently homosexual orientation but also his sociopolitical support of gay rights. Is it wrong for health-care professionals to express their values online in this way? I would say no. While each of us has a professional identity, we also have a personal identity as individuals who belong to ethnic groups, sexual minority groups, political groups, and so on. We are entitled to express our views and values online as individuals. So when do we need to disclose our personal affiliations and values to our patients? This is a trickier issue that calls into play the patient's right to know versus the professional's right to privacy. In the gay pediatrician example, the pediatrician would seem to have a right to hold private his own sexual orientation; he was "outed" by the online newspaper. However, if the pediatrician's sexual orientation begins to play a role in the treatment, for example if he becomes attracted to the young male patient, then the conflict will need to be managed – although not online.

In this day and age in which health care is front and center of the political arena, health-care professionals may feel motivated to become activists. They may do so in part out of the wish to advocate for what they perceive as the best interest of patients. Thus, they may support specific legislative initiatives or write letters to the editor of the local paper expressing an opinion about various aspects of health care. This kind of support may well be discoverable online as well. Is such advocacy inherently wrong? Should health-care professionals abstain from this kind of political involvement? To do so would be disrespectful of their own rights and arguably do a disservice to patients who need us as public advocates. However, we do need to disclose our professional identities when we take a public political stand, online or otherwise.

The issue of conflict of interest has been particularly "hot" in health-care research and academia in recent years, thanks to media coverage of events that highlight it. For example, in 2007 the commission of the Food and Drug Administration in the United States pleaded guilty to filing false reports regarding share ownership in pharmaceutical companies and was fined \$90,000 (Yen, 2009). At Harvard Medical School, medical students in a pharmacology class took action with administration after a faculty member ridiculed a student who appeared critical of a group of medications known as statins, and it turned out the faculty member had undisclosed ties with the pharmaceutical industry (Wilson, 2009). With the advent of online research – subjects being recruited and even treated over the Internet – the need for attention to conflict of interest is heightened. In the case of research, not only is there a potential conflict between the patients/subjects' wellbeing and the self-interest of the investigator (who may stand to gain professionally, academically, and even monetarily from the research), a potential conflict also exists between the investigator's private interest and the duty to maintain the integrity of the science. Guidelines that attempt to delineate appropriate interactions between investigators and industry sponsors, as well as guidelines that stipulate how funding should be disclosed to research subjects as part of the informed consent, apply in the online setting as well (Chimonas & Rothman, 2005).

7.4 GENERAL RECOMMENDATIONS FOR MANAGING CONFLICTS OF INTEREST ONLINE

How should conflicts of interest be managed? The safest way is to avoid conflicting roles. Health-care professionals should avoid taking on secondary roles that place them in clear conflict with their primary role. Sometimes this avoidance means not taking on conflicting responsibilities; for example, the clinical head of a hospital medical service should probably not also be the person who leads that hospital's online fundraising efforts. Sometimes conflicts are temporary and can be managed by not participating in a particular situation. For example, it is not uncommon for health-care professionals to develop medical products or write books. In such situations they should avoid endorsing any such product on online reviewing sites or being involved in financial decisions that affect it, such as its endorsement by a professional organization to which they belong (e.g. the American Medical Association).

Technology can pose a problem in terms of role separation. For example, many online companies including Facebook provide a service in exchange for advertising. The user of the site may have little control over what advertisements "pop up" on his or her site. And online companies collect information precisely to best identify what products would be most of interest to the site user. Thus, a health-care professional who uses Facebook might find that certain pharmaceuticals are advertising on his page without the professional having any knowledge or control. The contiguous placement of the advertisement may suggest an endorsement, or observers of the site may infer an endorsement, regardless of whether such an endorsement is intended.

If participation in a conflicting role cannot be avoided, full disclosure of the potential conflict to all those involved, and especially to those who stand to be harmed by any conflict, may be the next best solution. In general the maxim is that when in doubt whether a conflict exists, it is preferable to err on the side of disclosure. Obtaining consultation can also be helpful by providing a, hopefully, more distant and clearer perspective on what the underlying issues of the conflict might be and in identifying all the potential players who may be affected.

Limit setting is a strategy that refers to reducing the amount of gain that may potentially be had through the private interest of the activity. For example, a health-care professional who develops a product that makes money may decide to contribute the revenue to not-for-profit ventures that support patients. Some institutions set limits on how much practitioners can gain financially from relationships with the private sector.

Diversification may also be helpful in reducing any overdependence by the professional on sources of gain. For example, if a nurse practitioner (NP) blogs in a positive way about a certain antihypertensive and the manufacturer then offers to provide free samples to the clinic where the NP works, that person may also want to reach out to other manufacturers in a similar way to avoid the reality or the appearance of a preferential relationship.

Fundamental to the avoidance and management of real and potential conflicts of interest is the need for ongoing monitoring of one's own behavior. Increasingly, professional institutions are establishing oversight bodies for this purpose. Conflict of interest policies are explicitly delineating expectations and appear to be most effective when consequences for policy violations are also spelled out and enforced.

CONCLUSION

Conflict of interest is a complicated ethical and professionalism area and the advent of the Internet and digital technology has magnified how complicated it is. The first step is awareness of the issue and the ability to identify potential conflicts. The importance of not posting online content anonymously should be underscored. If we as health-care professionals are going to express a professional opinion online or advocate for any cause, including our own financial gain, we need to identify ourselves and our professional role. In the years to come, health-care and academic medical institutions are likely to develop guidelines for the appropriate use of the Internet in this regard.

REFERENCES

Chimonas, S., & Rothman, D. S. (2005). New federal guidelines for physician–pharmaceutical industry relations: The politics of policy formation. *Health Affairs*, *24*(4), 949–960. Retrieved from <http://content.healthaffairs.org/content/24/4/949.full>.

Gabbard, G. O., Roberts, L. W., Crisp-Han, J., Ball, V., Hobday, G., & Rachal, F. (2012). Overlapping roles and conflict of interest: *Professionalism in psychiatry*. Washington, DC: American Psychiatric Press. pp. 115–129.

Gregory, J. (1772). *Lectures on the duties and qualifications of a physician*. London, England: W. Strahan & T. Caddell.

Lagu, T., Kaufman, E. J., Asch, D. A., & Armstrong, K. (2008). Content of weblogs written by health professionals. *Journal of General Internal Medicine*, *23*, 1642–1646.

IOM (Institute of Medicine). (2009). *Conflict of interest in medical research, education and practice*. Washington, DC: National Academies Press.

Relman, A. S. (2007). The problem of commercialism in medicine. *Cambridge Quarterly of Healthcare Ethics*, *16*, 375–376.

Wilson, D. (2009). Harvard Medical School in ethics quandary. *The New York Times*, March 3.

Yen, H. (2009). FDA ex-chief spared jail time. *Washington Times*, February. 28. Retrieved from <http://washingtontimes.com.metro> via <http://bit.ly/103AIgO>.

Chapter | Eight

Academic Honesty

Why is academic honesty an important topic for health-care professionals? Of course, it has direct relevance to those who are also academicians, be they teachers, researchers, academic administrators, or all of the above. In that context, academic honesty is an important aspect of professionalism: The integrity of the academic work is central to the integrity of the professional. But the reality is that all of us in health care rely on information in order to help patients, and the integrity of that information is central to its quality.

The digital age has brought with it an exponential rise in the amount of accessible information. As University of North Carolina Professor Oliver Smithies, who won the Nobel Prize in 2007 for work in genetics he started at Oxford in 1947, is quoted as saying, "[T]he biggest change between then and now is the huge amount of information that is available" (Stafford, 2010, p. S19). According to a special report in *The Economist*, the volume of digital data now exceeds a zettabyte (10^{21}), equal to 35 trillion gigabytes (2010). The growth in online information is in part due to the ease of making information accessible. As *Nature* writer Ned Stafford points out: "Scientists are able to bypass traditional publication routes by quickly and easily posting academic papers, scientific data and personal blogs on the Internet." "Stafford notes that this ease of access has facilitated plagiarism:" Cheats have never had it so easy, able to copy and paste others' electronic information with little more than a mouse-click and claim it as their own" (Stafford, 2010, S19–20). And so the term "mouse-click plagiarism" has been coined (Auer & Krupar, 2001).

At the same time, digital technology and the Internet have allowed a much more systematic approach to discovering plagiarism. Harold Skip Garner, head of the Virginia Bioinformatics Institute at Virginia Tech, has developed online search engines to

S. deJong: Blogs and Tweets, Texting and Friending.
DOI: http://dx.doi.org/10.1016/B978-0-12-408128-4.00008-4
© 2014 S. DeJong. Published by Elsevier Inc. All rights reserved.

detect plagiarism, including eTBLAST. Stafford quotes Garner: "In the recent past, that is only two to three years ago, most plagiarism discoveries were serendipitous. But now they are being discovered en masse using computer techniques" (Stafford, 2010, p. S20).

The Office of Research Integrity of the U.S. Department of Health and Human Services offers the following definition of plagiarism: "The taking of words, images, ideas etc. from an author and presenting them as one's own. It is often associated with phrases, such as kidnapping of ideas, fraud, and literary theft" (Roig, n.d.). Academic institutions may have policies against plagiarism, including sanctions, but no laws govern plagiarism. Copyright infringement, on the other hand, is a legal concept pertaining to the creation, distribution, and reproduction of original work. When copyrighted material is used or copied without permission, even with proper citation, copyright laws may be broken and potential sanctions include fines and imprisonment (Dames, 2007, p. 24).

Evidence suggests that mouse-click plagiarism is on the rise. Donald McCabe, Professor of Management and Global Business at Rutgers University, has systematically studied plagiarism by surveying students and faculty since 1990 (McCabe, Trevino, & Butterfield, 2001; McCabe, n.d). Using web-based surveys of undergraduates, graduate students, and faculty, McCabe has worked through the Academic Integrity Assessment Project based at Duke University's Center for Academic Integrity to get a "pulse" of academic integrity on university campuses. In a recent survey of 63,700 undergraduates, 36% reported paraphrasing or copying a few sentences from an Internet source without footnoting it; of 9,250 graduate students, 25% reported such plagiarism; and of 9,000 faculty members, 69% reported such activity (McCabe, undated, pp. 6–7). These rates are actually lower than the reported rates by the same groups of plagiarizing from written sources. McCabe attributes this finding in part to some confusion as to what each question is asking: Does cutting and pasting from an online article mean taking it from a "written source" or from the Internet?

These same respondents appeared to recognize that such activities constituted moderate or serious cheating: In all three groups, 90–100% of respondents answered that turning in written work that was either copied from or done by another student was cheating. However, when asked about paraphrasing or copying a few sentences from an Internet source without footnoting it, responses were less robust. Over 40% of undergraduates, 30% of graduate students, and almost 20% of faculty were not convinced that "cut-and-paste plagiarism" is either moderate or serious cheating (McCabe et al., 2001).

A study by Scanlon and Neumann conducted in 1999–2000 looked specifically at Internet plagiarism rates among 698 college students. The pencil-and-paper study asked about cutting and pasting, soliciting papers from others, and purchasing papers from online term paper mills. In their sample, 24.5% of students reported plagiarizing online; some reported doing so very frequently. Interestingly, respondents estimated that their peers plagiarized from online sources much more frequently than they did: Respondents guessed that up to 50% of their peers had engaged in copying text without a citation (Scanlon & Neumann, 2002, p. 383). This data may suggest that online plagiarism is less common than the respondents believed; however, McCabe and colleagues have concluded that "peer-related contextual factors," which include perceptions of peer behavior, are strongly associated with student behavior. Thus, if most students believe their colleagues are plagiarizing from online sources, they may be more likely to do it themselves.

In his book *The Shadow Scholar: How I Made a Living Helping College Kids Cheat,* Dave Tomar (2010) reports earning $66,000 a year working as a writer-for-hire for college students. He describes ghost-writing personal statements, term papers, and even one doctoral dissertation, often with the full knowledge of the student's parents (Demeron, 2012). In 2002 Turnitin.com, a plagiarism-detection service, reported having 400 client colleges in the US (Foster, 2002, A37), and the Canadian Broadcasting Corporation reported in 2005 that Turnitin had 4,000 students using its services (cited in Howard, 2007). One study by researchers at Duquesne University found that the more online tools college students were permitted to use in completing an assignment, the more likely they were to copy the work of others (Perez-Pena, 2012).

Few surveys of plagiarism in health-care professional schools exist. However, cheating expert McCabe has studied this issue and completed a survey of nursing students in 2007 (McCabe, 2009). He cited earlier studies by Hilbert (1987) and Bailey (1990), as well as a survey by Brown (2002) in which it was reported that of 253 nursing students, more than 75% reported having seen another student cheat and 17% reported having cheated themselves. In his own study of over a thousand nursing students, McCabe found that 36% undergraduate respondents reported copying "a few sentences from a Web source without citing it" and 22% of graduate nursing students reported the same. In more recent surveys, McCabe reports finding that "87% of nursing students indicated that the Internet was the exclusive or primary mechanism they used to access plagiarized material." McCabe concludes:

> *Although the Internet has become the mechanism of choice,*
> *it is less clear whether it has led to a dramatic increase*
> *in the number of students who plagiarize. Anecdotal*
> *evidence from both faculty and students, both nursing and*

non-nursing, suggests that those who plagiarize using the Internet plagiarize with greater frequency than those still relying on written copying. This difference appears to be based on the ease with which they can access the desired material and the time saved as a result ... Although one may argue that the Internet has not led to a dramatic increase in the number of students who plagiarize, it does seem to have led to a dramatic increase in the amount of minor, or cut-and-paste, plagiarism that occurs.

McCabe, 2009, p. 619

Another survey in 2011 by psychologist Dora D. Clarke-Pine at La Sierra University in Riverside, CA, found that of 120 doctoral dissertations submitted by psychology students in a nationwide sample, 80% contained examples of 10 or more words of word-for-word plagiarism (Cohen, 2011). Whether the source of the plagiarized words was online or from elsewhere is not revealed.

An area in which plagiarism has been a concern is in the application process to graduate medical education. However, no systematic studies exist and findings are largely anecdotal. For example, one family medicine program in Florida found that of 26 applications to their program over a two-year period, three of the personal statements contained sections that were plagiarized from the same website (Cole, 2007). An online search finds plenty of online sites in which personal statements for medical students can be located (see, for example, http://www.medfools.com/personal-statements.php).

Some academicians have argued that online text lacks access controls and thus is more subject to abuse. For example, Enos and Borrowman (2001, p. 95) argue:

The Internet does not have the controls placed on it that traditional media, such as television and print, do. In such an open forum, traditional notions of authorship and ethos are challenged. And when there is challenge, the temptation is to retreat into tradition, into the comfortable world of the known-and-familiar.

Others have argued that the increased availability of new texts is simply an opportunity for our culture to revise its thinking about textuality (Howard, 2007). A case in point is the award-winning novel *Axolotl Roadkill* by 17-year-old Helene Hegemann whose book was shown to be plagiarized from an online blog and other sources including a novel, *Strobo*. In *The New York Times*, the author is reported as having "apologized for not being more open about her sources, ... [but] also defended herself as the representative of a different generation, one that freely mixes and matches from the whirring flood of information across new and old media, to create something new." In a statement, Ms. Hegemann allegedly added: "There's no such thing as originality anyway, just authenticity" (Kulish, 2012).

Stories like these raise the question of whether the concepts "intellectual property" and "authorship" are being defined in a fundamentally different way by "digital natives," those under the age of 30, who grew up in the digital age and many of whom argue for completely open access to intellectual material. (Their current icon is Aaron Swartz, a Harvard Fellow who committed suicide in 2013 after facing prosecution for downloading subscription-based documents from MIT's online library system.) The Internet provides a free, open-access platform for everything from wikis (like Wikipedia) to software such as Linux. Wiki communities and other online collaborations have spawned innovation such as the Human Genome Project. Crowdsourcing, the process of acquiring services, ideas or content by soliciting a large group, such as an online community, moves ownership of intellectual content from the individual to the "crowd" (Topol, 2012, pp. 9–12).

Like the concept of privacy discussed earlier (see Chapter 5), "originality" and "intellectual property" may be in the process of being redefined, as Ms. Hegemann's statement suggests. Academicians point to examples such as a student at DePaul University who presented a paper to his writing tutor with large sections in purple text. The purple sections were downloaded from the Web. When confronted by the tutor, the student allegedly did not see anything wrong and did not become defensive; he simply wanted help in turning the text from purple to black (Gabriel, 2010). Another student cited in the same *New York Times* story allegedly plagiarized from Wikipedia and when disciplined explained that since the entries were "unsigned and collectively written" they were "common knowledge." As Teresa Fishman, director of the Center for Academic Integrity at Clemson University, is quoted by *The New York Times* as saying: "Now we have a whole generation of students who've grown up with information that just seems to be hanging out there in cyberspace and doesn't seem to have an author. It's possible to believe this information is just out there for anyone to take." Ms. Fishman's observation seems to be supported by McCabe's research, which has found that the percentage of respondents to his surveys who believe that copying from the Web represents serious cheating is actually falling (McCabe, n.d.).

Anthropologist Susan D. Blum, author of *My Word! Plagiarism and College Culture* (2009), argues that traditions such as original work belonging to the individual and intellectual property rights being guarded by copyright law are traditions being challenged in the current digital culture. "Our notion of authorship and originality was born, it flourished, and it may be waning," Ms. Blum is quoted as saying in *The New York Times* (Gabriel, 2010).

Whatever may be happening in the world of art and fiction, in the world of science and health care, plagiarism – online and otherwise – remains an academic offense subject to discipline. A Google search of "plagiarism" turns up numerous private entities which sponsor online plagiarism detection services, some of which (such as plagiarism.org) are free. Here, the permanence of the Internet may prove useful: As editors of *Medical Hypotheses*, an online journal, write:

> *Many writers and researchers are reluctant to publish online for fear that their work will be plagiarized and used without attribution elsewhere … However, if this happens, plagiarism may be objectively proven by a service called the Internet Archive Wayback Machine (archive.org). Archive.org permits clarification of the issue of dates – and allows the reader to draw their own conclusions about authorship, whether charitable or otherwise.*
>
> **Medical Hypotheses, 2009**

What is the impact of online plagiarism? The individual whose work is plagiarized certainly feels violated, as Stanley Fish attests in his *New York Times* blog (Fish, 2010). Fish described how, as a college dean, he discovered that two scholars on his faculty had apparently copied two pages from one of his books and placed it in their own. When confronted, one co-author allegedly responded that he had not written that one. On contacting the co-author he was told "something about graduate student researchers who had given him material that was not properly identified." Fish (2010) concludes:

> *Whether there is something called originality or not, the two scholars who began their concluding chapter by reproducing two of my pages are professionally culpable. They took something from me without asking and without acknowledgment, and they profited – if only in the currency of academic reputation – from work that I had done and signed. That's the bottom line, and no fancy philosophical argument can erase it.*

The more rampant plagiarism becomes, the more foundations of scientific knowledge may come into question. An issue of the journal *Nature*, for example, described frequent occurrences of plagiarism among political figures in Europe, including Germany's former defense minister Karl-Theodor zu Guttenberg and Romania's prime minister Victor Ponta, both accused of plagiarism in their law theses, and Hungary's former president Paul Schmitt, who allegedly incorporated plagiarized material into his physical education thesis. In addition to the negative impact on academia caused by promoting the careers of "the fraudulent and the undeserving" and imbuing students with "disrespect for scientific method and academic principles," the editors suggest a larger-scale impact, pointing to Romania as an example:

> *Most countries accept that to attain economic prosperity*
> *they need a robust research base, a concept enshrined in*
> *the European Union's Treaty of Lisbon. But a research base*
> *contaminated with plagiarism can never function optimally.*
> *Romania, a signatory to the treaty, seemed to be on track*
> *to a more honest and promising future when it passed*
> *its education law, designed to inject competition into its*
> *universities and root out widespread scientific misconduct.*
> *Yet that law is now being undermined by political*
> *interference in the very ethics councils that should be helping*
> *to implement it. Against this backdrop, it is easy to see why*
> *Romania's excellent scientists – and there are many of them –*
> *choose to work mostly outside the country.*
>
> **Nature, 2012**

Efforts are underway to educate about the plagiarism problem. In Romania, a group of researchers is using a website to track and investigate cases of scientific misconduct. In the United States, education efforts are evident in ventures such as *The New York Times* The Learning Network (Dekorne & Khan, 2003). Research librarians and others affiliated with academic programs have developed innovative methods to teach plagiarism awareness (Glassman, Sorensen, Habousha, Minuti, & Schwartz, 2011; Lowe & Stone, 2010). The Department of Health and Human Services' Office of Research Integrity has published a guide to avoiding plagiarism (Roig, n.d.).

8.1 VIGNETTES

To understand the potential role of plagiarism and other aspects of academic misconduct in health care, let us look at some vignettes.

Vignette 8.1

A psychologist attends a conference and hears a presentation by a colleague on the topic of personality disorders. The speaker presents a case. As she listens, the psychologist increasingly recognizes the content of the case presentation: It is a verbatim copy from a case she had written about and published, with the patient's permission, in an open-access journal. The psychologist feels angry that her work has been stolen and is now being represented as the work of someone else. She also feels angry on behalf of the patient, who had not given consent for the case to be presented in a conference. The psychologist is not sure how to proceed.

Here we can identify with the psychologist's feeling of being violated – not unlike that of having one's home broken into by burglars. Not only has something been taken in this case, but someone else is now flaunting it as his own. How should the psychologist proceed? Generally conferences, particularly those run by a professional association, have program committees who are responsible for upholding the integrity of the content. The psychologist's concerns should be brought to the chair of the program committee. Why take action at all? The failure of the psychologist to take action may result in the presenter continuing to engage in dishonest academic behavior out of the belief that he can get away with it.

Vignette 8.2

A multi-site, randomized-controlled trial of a widely used, relatively new medication to treat hypertension is published in a prestigious journal which is also available online and indexed on major medical databases. The study finds the medication has a moderate effect size and, unlike general clinical experience with this medication, does not cause significant side-effects such as weight gain and headaches. In the months that follow publication, health-care-focused digital media include lively and excited discussion about these new findings. Some months after publication, an ethics complaint is filed with the editor of the journal that published the paper. The complaint claims that the data was falsified. Up to a year later, a retraction had not been published by the journal.

Falsification of data is certainly not a new issue in research and academia. What is different in the digital age is the rapid dissemination of information. The results of the study would have been widely communicated and imprinted on the minds of health-care professionals and the public alike. Conducting an inquiry into allegations of research impropriety can take a very long time and may not cause the same stir as the initial results. And what if there is a retraction? Health-care professionals who had been prescribing this medication and using this study as evidence in the informed consent process with patients are left in a difficult position.

As H. R. Garner, Professor and Director of the Medical Informatics and Systems Division at Virginia Bioinformatics Institute points out, published papers with academic integrity concerns "continue to be unwittingly used by professionals to make scientific, even clinical decisions. Even after questionable documents have been identified, judged, and retracted, that retraction notice may never propagate back to the indexing and search services" (Garner, 2011, p. 95). Garner looked at similar pairs of manuscripts in 1,000 papers on Medline that were deposited in the Déjà vu database and found that a decline occurred in suspected duplicates from 2006 to 2008 (p. 96). He noted that the number of retractions had also increased, and attributed both changes in part to the advent of plagiarism detection services. But, importantly, he concluded: "The plagiarism detection services are working to intercept and deter future attempts at plagiarism, but what are we to do with all the plagiarized material that has been accumulating over time?" He noted the significant harm that results from plagiarism: "Scientists or clinicians can use the data to make research or patient judgments that are wrong, editors and reviewers use their valuable time to review these manuscripts, and the lay public questions the quality of science and medicine when public revelations of misbehavior surface" (p. 95). Patients need to be informed about the retraction of the previously held findings; however, doing so is an embarrassment to the prescriber and the profession.

8.2 GENERAL RECOMMENDATIONS

What can you do if you suspect your own work has been plagiarized? As mentioned above, a number of different software programs for plagiarism detection have been developed. Most simply, a sample from the text can be cut and pasted into the search box on Google, Google Scholar, Medline, PubMed Central, and Wikipedia. A company called iParadigms, LLC offers two services: TurnItIn (http://turnitin.com) is for use by academic institutions, and iThenticate (http://www.ithenticate.com), which works with the citation-linking software CrossRef (the not-for-profit company that developed Digital Object Identifiers for citations), is for publishers and researchers (Glassman, Sorensen, Habousha, Minuti & Schwartz, 2011). Another software (eTBLAST from Virginia Tech, http://etest.vbi.vt.edu/etblast3/) is a search engine for similar text that was developed to detect plagiarism. However, as in Vignette 8.2, even when plagiarism or other academic falsifications are detected, many papers and documents that have ethical issues remain online.

Advice on coping with online plagiarism is available, of course, online. Authors at plagiarismtoday.com discuss confronting the plagiarist and, if this fails, telling the website host about the plagiarism. Typically websites are hosted by people or companies called internet service providers (ISPs). On each website there is a URL at the top of the browser. A typical URL format is http://subdomain.domain.extension/folder. The subdomain is typically "www" and the extension is typically "org" or "com" or "net." For example, in http://www.medicalblog.com/xxxxx, the domain is medicalblog. Locating the host can also be achieved using services such as WhoIsHostingThis (WiHT) and pasting the domain in to the lookup box (www.plagiarismtoday.com/stopping-internet-plagiarism/3-finding-the-host/).

CONCLUSION

Academic honesty, like so many of the core topics in this book, is not a new concern. However, once again, the Internet and digital technology offer a new dimension to the problem: "Mouse-click" plagiarism seems to have permeated the world of science, including health care. Plagiarism and lack of scholarly integrity are not only an academic concern, however; the integrity of scientific research and disseminated scholarship are fundamental to the reliability of health-care information that we apply to patients every day.

Mouse-click plagiarism may be only the beginning. The facility with which especially brief content can be cut and pasted has made the practice so routine that it has blurred the boundaries of intellectual property that have traditionally defined academic content. Original work that is a pastiche of the work of others may be viewed as acceptable by digital natives.

The Internet has now entered the world of scientific research, in terms of methodology, and the Association of Internet Researchers (http://aoir.com) was founded to focus on these issues. Research studies routinely recruit subjects from online sources. Some research studies are largely conducted through online exchange of information. In 2011, the FDA approved the first-ever randomized "virtual" clinical trial: In the REMOTE study (Research on Electronic Monitoring of OAC Treatment Experience), researchers at Pfizer started using mobile phones, YouTube, and other web-based technologies to allow patients with overactive bladder (OAB) to participate in a study to assess the safety and efficacy of tolterodine tartrate. Approximately 600 subjects from 10 states across the USA were slated to participate (www.pharmafile.com via http://bit.ly/17e2tJY).

Other researchers use the Internet to study subjects. For example, Moreno et al. (2009) identified at-risk adolescents using their MySpace profiles and made online interventions regarding sexual and substance abuse behaviors. The ethical complexities of such research abound: If these teenagers are minors, how is informed consent obtained? To what extent can data be collected about these adolescents' "friends"? (Shapiro & Ossorio, 2013). (For more information about Internet research, see www.hhs.gov via http://1.usa.gov/11vHGz5).

In summary, the academic domain, like that of clinical care, faces unprecedented challenges in the digital age. Health-care professionals will do well to move quickly to take a leadership role in how things should move forward, rather than being in a position of racing to keep up.

REFERENCES

Auer, N. J., & Krupar, E. M. (2001). Mouse-click plagiarism: The role of technology in plagiarism and the librarian's role in combating it. *Library Trends*, *49*(3), 415–432.

Bailey, P. A. (1990). Cheating among nursing students. *Nurse Educator*, *15*(3), 32–35.

Blum, S. D. (2009). *My Word! Plagiarism and college culture*. Cornell, NY: Cornell University Press.

Brown, D. L. (2002). Cheating must be okay. Everybody does it!. *Nurse Educator*, *27*, 608.

Cohen, P. (2011). Thinking cap: The seemingly persistent rise of plagiarism. *The New York Times,* Aug 23. Retrieved from <artsbeat.blogs.nytimes.com>.

Cole, A. F. (2007). Plagiarism in graduate medical education. *Family Medicine*, *29*(6), 436–438.

Dames, R. K. (2007). Understanding plagiarism and how it differs from copyright infringement. *Computers in Libraries*, *27*, 6.

Dekorne, C. & Khan, J. (2003). Please no posers. Lesson plan. The learning network. Retrieved from <http://learning.blogs.nytimes.com/2003/09/04/please-no-posers/>.

Demeron, C. (2012). A man for all semesters. *The Wall Street Journal*, September 2.

Enos, T., & Borrowman, S. (2001). Authority and credibility: Classical rhetoric, the Internet, and the teaching of techno-ethos. In L. Gray-Rosendale

& S. Gruber (Eds.), *Alternative rhetorics: Challenges to the rhetorical tradition (pp. 93–110)*. Carbondale: Southern Illinois UP.

Fish, S. (2010). Plagiarism is not a big moral deal. *The New York Times*. Retrieved from <opininator.blogs.nytimes.com/2010>.

Foster, A.L. (2002). Plagiarism detection tool creates legal quandary. *The Chronicle of Higher Education*, May 17.

Gabriel, T. (2010). Plagiarism lines blur for students in digital age. *The New York Times*, August 1.

Garner, H. R. (2011). Combating unethical publications with plagiarism detection services. *Urologic Oncology*, *29*, 95–99.

Glassman, N. R., Sorensen, K., Habousha, R. G., Minuti, A., & Schwartz, R. (2011). The plagiarism project. *Medical Reference Services Quarterly*, *30*(4), 337–348.

Hilbert, G. A. (1987). Academic fraud: Prevalence, practice and reasons. *Journal of Professional Nursing*, *3*, 39–45.

Howard, R. M. (2007). Understanding "internet plagiarism". *Computers and Composition*, *24*, 3–15.

Kulish, N. (2012). Author, 17, says it's 'mixing,' not plagiarism. *The New York Times*, Feb 11.

Lowe, S. M., & Stone, S. M. (2010). Information literacy for professional programs: Two case studies at one university. *Information Outlook*, *14*(6), 17.

McCabe, D. L., (n.d.). Cheating among college and university students: a North American perspective. *International Journal for Educational Integrity*. Retrieved from <http://www.ojs.unisa.edu.au/index.php/IJEI/article/viewFile/14/9>.

McCabe, D. L. (2009). Academic dishonesty in nursing schools: An empirical investigation. *Journal of Nursing Education*, *48*(11), 614–623. http://dx.doi.org/10.3928/0148834-20090716-07.

McCabe, D. L., Trevino, L. K., & Butterfield, K. D. (2001). Cheating in academic institutions: A decade of research. *Ethics and Behavior*, *11*(3), 219–232.

Medical Hypotheses (2009). Editorial: Plagiarism of online material may be proven using the Internet Archive Wayback Machine (archive.org). *Medical Hypotheses*, *73*, 875.

Moreno, M. A., VanderStoep, A., Parks, M. R., Zimmerman, F. J., Kurth, A., & Christakis, D. A. (2009). Display of health risk behaviors on MySpace by adolescents: prevalence and associations. *Archives of Pediatric and Adolescent Medicine*, *163*(1), 27–34. http://dx.doi.org/10.1001/archpediatrics.2008.528.

Nature (2012). Editorial: Repeat after me. *Nature*, *488*, 253.

Perez-Pena R. (2012). Studies find more students cheating with high achievers no exception. *The New York Times*, September 7.

Roig, M. (n.d.). Avoiding plagiarism. Self-plagiarism and other questionable writing practices: A guide to ethical writing. Office of Research Integrity, U.S. Department of Health and Human Services. Retrieved from <http://ori.dhhs.gov/education/products/plagiarism/>.

Scanlon, P. M., & Neumann, D. R. (2002). Internet plagiarism among college students. *Journal of College Student Development*, *43*(3), 374–385.

Shapiro, R. B., & Ossorio, P. N. (2013). Regulation of online social network studies. *Science*, *339*, 144–145.

Siegele, L. (2010). It's a smart world; special report on smart systems. November 4, 2010. *The Economist*. Retrieved from <www.economist.com/node/17388368>.

Stafford, N. (2010). Science in the digital age. *Nature*, *467*, S19–S21.

Tomar, D. (2010). The shadow scholar: How I made a living helping college kids cheat: *New York*. Bloomsbury, USA.

Topol, E. (2012). *The creative destruction of medicine – How the digital revolution will create better health care*. New York: Basic Books.

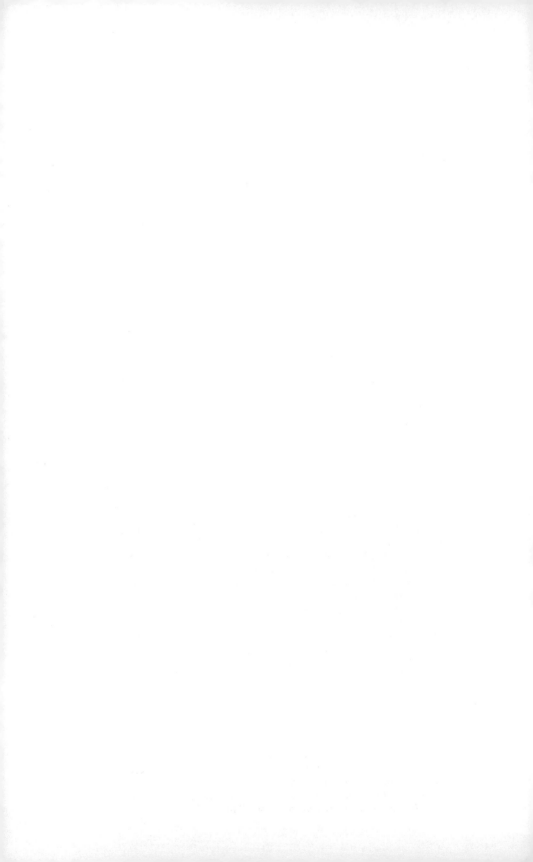

Chapter Nine

Mandated Reporting and Safety Issues

As health-care professionals, we have a role in protecting not only our patients but also vulnerable members of our society and, in some circumstances, society as a whole. In many democratic societies, the law mandates that physicians and other health-care professionals report suspected abuse or neglect of vulnerable individuals. "Vulnerable" is defined differently in different jurisdictions, but generally refers to minors (children and adolescents), the elderly, and the disabled. Some jurisdictions require the reporting of suspected domestic violence as well. Other mandated reported requirements focus on potential impairment of health-care professionals themselves. For example, medical licensing boards may require that professional peers report on each other if impairment due to an issue such as substance abuse is suspected. Other laws emphasize a public health concern: Laws may require medical professionals to report potentially impaired patients who may endanger others; one such example is alcoholic patients who may be at risk of harming members of the public by driving while intoxicated. And finally, many public health systems require reporting of infectious and communicable diseases such as HIV and syphilis.

9.1 HEALTH-CARE PROFESSIONALS' DUTY TO PROTECT

Society's duty to protect children dates back to the seventeenth century. John Locke argued that the right of parental guardianship was contingent upon it being appropriately exercised, and that it could be taken away if it was not (Locke, 2003; cited in Mathew & Bross, 2008). In the nineteenth century, at the height of the industrial revolution, John Stuart Mill lobbied for the protection of children from

S. deJong: Blogs and Tweets, Texting and Friending.
DOI: http://dx.doi.org/10.1016/B978-0-12-408128-4.00009-6
© 2014 S. DeJong. Published by Elsevier Inc. All rights reserved.

external harm and argued that the family was the most important domain in which the state should be able to intervene to prevent the abuse of power (Mill, 1998). Parents remain the most common perpetrators, and they in general do not pursue help themselves. In 2004 in the United States, according to the U.S. Dept of Health and Human Services (HSS) only 0.1% of abuse reports were made by the alleged perpetrators and another 4% by nonperpetrating parents (HSS, 2006).

Although mandated reporting remains controversial and problematic in terms of if and how reports are investigated, evidence suggests that mandated reporting does increase substantiated and unsubstantiated referrals to child protective services. Mandated reporting laws (together with investigation and treatment services) are estimated to have resulted in a decline in annual child deaths from between 3,000 and 5,000 to about 1,100 in the United States (Besharov, 1985, p. 287). Evidence about the importance of preventing child maltreatment keeps mounting (Shonkoff, Boyce, & McEwen, 2009).

Who is a mandated reporter varies between jurisdictions. In the United States, child protection laws vary by state. The state of Vermont, generally considered politically liberal, requires health-care providers, school staff, employers of human service agencies, police and probation officers, camp personnel, and members of the clergy to report if there is a "reasonable cause to believe that a child has been abused or neglected" (HSS, 2010, p. 49). The state of Texas, a more conservative state traditionally, requires that teachers, daycare employees, "nurses, doctors, or employees of a clinical or health-care facility that provides reproductive services," and "juvenile probation officers or juvenile detention or correctional officers" report if they have cause to believe that a child has been adversely affected by abuse or neglect" (HSS, 2010, p. 48).

The laws to protect children have been expanded in more recent years to cover other potentially vulnerable individuals. Some states, for example California, Colorado, Kentucky, and New Hampshire, require health-care workers to report domestic violence (Iavicolli, 2005). Other laws protect the physically and mentally disabled and the elderly. Some laws cover broad categories of who should be protected and from what. For example, in Minnesota, a vulnerable adult is an 18-year-old or older who:

- is a resident or inpatient of a facility OR
- receives services from an adult service facility OR
- receives services from a home care provider or personal care assistant OR
- regardless of receiving services, possesses a physical, mental, or emotional infirmity or dysfunction that impairs the person's ability to provide adequately for his/her own care without assistance AND
- has an impaired ability to protect him/herself from maltreatment.

Abuse can include: assault; use of drugs to injure or facilitate a crime; solicitation, inducement or promotion of prostitution; sexual conduct that meets the elements of a crime; hitting, slapping, kicking, pinching, biting, or corporal punishment; use of repeated or malicious oral, written or gestured language that would be considered disparaging, humiliating, or threatening; use of unauthorized aversive or deprivation procedures, unreasonable confinement, or involuntary seclusion; sexual contact or penetration between facility staff and client; forcing or coercing to perform services for another's advantages" (Sexual Violence Justice Institute, 2006).

In addition to protecting their patients, health-care professionals may have a duty to protect others from potential harm by their patients. The Tarasoff standard, based on a 1976 case, *Tarasoff v. Regents of the University of California*, requires psychiatrists and mental health clinicians who know or ought to know that specific persons may be at risk of harm by one of their patients to take reasonable steps to protect those persons (Appelbaum & Gutheil, 2007, p. 121). In some jurisdictions, including the province of Ontario in Canada, physicians are required to report patients who may be unfit to drive for medical reasons (Redelmeier, Vinkatesh & Stanbrook, 2008). In the state of Oregon, this requirement applies to mandated reporting of intoxicated driving (McManus, Magaret, Hedges, Rayner & Rice, 2005). Finally, many medical professions have a peer-reporting standard. In the state of Massachusetts, for example, the Board of Registration in Medicine (BRM) requires all health-care providers (including doctors, nurses, and psychologists) to report to the Board if they have a "reasonable basis" for concern that a physician is practicing medicine while impaired by drugs or alcohol, or uses drugs and/or alcohol regularly.[1]

In all of these laws, semantics are subject to interpretation. What is a "reasonable basis"? What constitutes a "reasonable cause to suspect" abuse? Evidence suggests that this language is interpreted in very different ways in practice and is subject to bias. For example, one study of child abuse found "no consensus in how experts on child abuse interpret 'reasonable suspicion'" (Levi & Crowell, 2011). Another study surveyed 532 visiting nurses across the United States regarding attitudes and behaviors regarding mandated reporting of partner violence. The study found a correlation between support of mandated reporting requirements regarding partner violence and the likelihood of reporting (Davidov, Nadorff, Jack, Coben, & NFP IPV Research Team, 2012).

So far, this discussion has focused on legal requirements, obviously an important part of professionalism. But, as discussed in

---

[1]Regulations of the Board of Registration in Medicine 243 Code of Massachusetts Regulations (CMR) 2.14.

Chapter 1, ethics are also an important aspect of professionalism, and some of our reporting requirements may be ethically as well as legally mandated; others may not meet the specific criteria of legal requirements, but nonetheless merit consideration on ethical grounds. As discussed in Chapter 1, ethical principles include the ethical obligation to do no harm. For example, if we know that someone under our care or known to us through our professional work is at risk of harming others, are we not ethically required to take action? And where do we draw the line?

9.2 SAFETY, MANDATED REPORTING, AND DIGITAL TECHNOLOGY

Into this already complicated legal and ethical landscape enters digital technology. As with so many areas of clinical practice, the Internet and current technology do not alter the conceptual foundation of mandated reporting requirements, but rather complicate them. By providing so many more ways for us to learn about patients and colleagues, technology can put us in the position of acquiring information, both inadvertently and intentionally, that may make us wonder whether we have a legal or ethical obligation to report the information to appropriate authorities.

Those health-care professionals working with youth, especially those with mental health issues, may be particularly likely to encounter a clinical decision point due to safety concerns expressed online. Not only can at-risk patients learn about how to commit suicide via online sources, they can also express their suicidality via various online and digital media and share suicide notes online (Baume, Cantor & Rolfe, 1997; Belfort, Mezzacappa & Ginnis, 2010).

9.2.1 Vignettes

Consider the following examples:

Vignette 9.1

An internist begins seeing a divorced, middle-aged male patient with various cardiac problems and depression. The patient is a celebrity in his academic field, but the internist is not very familiar with this field. In order to better understand his patient's expertise and academic stature, the physician googles the patient. The internist discovers signed blog entries on a number of different blogs, as well as the patient's Facebook site, in which the patient complains about his ex-girlfriends. In particular, the patient focuses on an ex-girlfriend who he feels humiliated him. In one of the entries, he makes reference to wanting to "kill the slut" and in another to wanting to "give her what she's asking for."

Adapted from DeJong et al., 2011, Vignette #13

Here, the physician has broken the treatment frame by searching online for information about his patient outside of a treatment session and without discussing the search first with the patient. The information he finds is problematic because it suggests that the patient has aggressive and even homicidal intentions towards a specific woman. This is an example of a health-care provider inadvertently learning information about a patient that is cause for concern. If the internist were a psychiatrist, the Tarasoff standard, if applicable in his jurisdiction, might require that the physician would need to take action to protect the identified woman from his aggressive patient. For this internist, the dilemma may be more ethical than legal. What is he now going to do with the information? Should he call the patient to express his concern? Should he tell the patient at the next visit? Should he not say anything to the patient and plan to make further assessment of the patient's risk for violence at the next visit? If he does disclose to the patient, how will the patient feel – angry, betrayed, violated, vengeful? Will the treatment relationship survive such a rupture?

This whole situation could have been averted if the internist had simply admitted to the patient that he was unaware of the patient's expertise but wanted to learn more about it. Could the patient refer the physician to some of his articles? Could he say more about his work? In this way, the treatment frame could have been preserved and the physician would have avoided potential charges of voyeurism. Of course, such an approach might have meant that the physician would not have learned, at least for now, about his patient's violent tendencies and the potential risk to the ex-girlfriend. If the risk is real and the physician is able to take action that protects the patient, one might argue that the break in the frame was offset by the safety benefit to the woman in question. In practical terms, the internist would do well to get legal, ethical, and clinical consultation regarding how best to proceed.

Let us consider a different vignette, this time pertaining to an adolescent patient.

Vignette 9.2

A pediatrician is treating an adolescent patient for abdominal pain and depression in the context of dysfunctional family dynamics, including a father with significant substance dependence. In a recent visit, the adolescent remarks that life at home was particularly difficult, but denies any frank abuse or neglect. The adolescent comments that she has been obtaining support from peers through her Facebook page. After the adolescent leaves the office, the pediatrician becomes concerned that the patient may have been minimizing the situation at home. The pediatrician looks up the adolescent's Facebook page and discovers multiple recent entries reporting that her father had been out of control, behaving like a "maniac," and swearing at and punching her mother. The patient describes on her web page being so afraid for herself that she wants to leave, but she does not want to abandon her younger siblings.

Adapted from DeJong et al., 2011, Vignette #14

Here again, the healthcare professional breaks the treatment frame and learns of a safety risk, this time involving the patient as potential victim of paternal violence. The frame break occurs in the context of an outpatient practice. However, because it pertains to the safety of children, the duty to protect may be clearer here. Again, the pediatrician would do well to get legal consultation. If the pediatrician does file a report with child protective services and the adolescent patient discovers that fact, the treatment alliance may be in jeopardy even though the pediatrician was acting in the best interest of the adolescent and her siblings. The outcome may well depend on whether the adolescent perceives the break in the frame as positive because it led to her family getting help, or whether she sees it as a violation of her privacy.

Let us look at one last example.

Vignette 9.3

An emaciated elderly woman is brought in to the emergency room by police after having been found wandering the streets in cold weather. The woman has no identification on her person, and can only recall her name but not her address nor any other details of her life. She remembers growing up in a local suburb. The emergency room team diagnoses dementia and the patient is treated for mild hypothermia and given IV fluids and food. Several hours later, the emergency room physician is ready to discharge the patient, but does not feel that it is safe to discharge her alone because she does not appear competent to take care of herself. The team searches hospital records and places calls to police, other emergency rooms, and local homeless shelters to see if anyone knows the patient. Finding no answers, the emergency room physician decides to go online. He googles the patient and finds an obituary in a local newspaper of a man with the patient's last name. In the obituary, the patient is identified as a sister of the deceased, and surviving relatives and their towns of residence are identified. The physician is then able to get in contact with a family member who can take the patient home.

In this case, too, the treatment frame is broken. However, the situation occurs in the emergency room (where certain rights such as confidentiality may be waived in order to provide appropriate care to the patient), and with a patient appears not to be competent to give consent to an online search. A risk–benefit analysis would seem to suggest that the physician took appropriate steps in searching about the patient online in order to safely discharge her from the emergency room.

9.3 GENERAL RECOMMENDATIONS

As these vignettes show, intentionally or unintentionally finding information about our patients that may raise safety issues and a duty to report can place the health-care professional in a difficult situation. The first recommendation is to stop and think before seeking information about a patient and, if something about a patient is found unexpectedly, stop and think before taking further action. For many health-care professionals in today's culture, online searching may be a reflexive habit – so normal in the course of their daily lives and done so quickly that they may miss the opportunity to think through the potential consequences of a search about a patient.

In general, it is preferable to respect the treatment frame. If the professional believes that information gained online may advance the patient's treatment, there is no harm in asking the patient whether they can go online together during a treatment visit. Together, they can share the information, thus preventing perceptions of curiosity or voyeurism.

If the information found raises safety concerns, the professional should seek legal, ethical, and clinical consultation regarding how best to proceed. Legal and ethical requirements may differ according to jurisdiction, medical specialty, and institution. As is often the case with these dilemmas, the adage that "the devil is in the details" often applies. While a legal and ethical resolution may rest with the duty to the patient, the patient may not always agree that the professional's actions were in his or her best interests, and difficult feelings may be elicited. The treatment alliance may not survive the process.

CONCLUSION

Health-care professionals may practice under legal, professional, and ethical obligations to report patients at risk of being harmed, harming themselves or harming others. Such obligations may particularly pertain to vulnerable populations such as children, the disabled, and the elderly and, for mental health professionals, the mentally ill. Technology provides a means for professionals to learn a great deal about patients' private lives. Professionals may learn of such information either by intentional online searches or inadvertently, through their own personal online activities. If this information raises safety concerns, the professional is faced with a difficult dilemma that transcends legal, ethical, professional, and clinical domains. Because of regional differences in mandated reporting requirements and the potential complexity of each case, professionals should pause before taking any action and consider obtaining excellent consultation.

REFERENCES

Appelbaum, P. S., & Gutheil, T. G. (2007). *Clinical handbook of psychiatry and the law*. Philadelphia: Wolters Kluwer/Lippincott Williams & Wilkins.

Baume, P., Cantor, C. H., & Rolfe, A. (1997). Cybersuicide: the role of interactive suicide notes on the Internet. *Crisis, 18*(2), 73–79.

Belfort, E., Mezzacappa, E. Ginnis K. (2010). Similarities and differences among adolescents who communicate suicidality via electronic versus other means. Poster presentation, American Academy of Child and Adolescent Psychiatry, October Annual Meeting.

Besharov, D. (1985). "Doing something" about child abuse: The need to narrow the grounds for state intervention. *Harvard Journal of Law and Public Policy, 8*(3) 359–389. p. 287.

Davidov, D. M., Nadorff, M. R., Jack, S. M., Coben, J., & NFP IPV Research Team. (2012). Nurse home visitors' perceptions of mandatory reporting of intimate partners violence to law enforcement agencies. *Journal of Interpersonal Violence, 27*(12), 2484–2502.

DeJong, S., et al. (2011). Curriculum on professionalism and the Internet. American Academy of Directors of Psychiatry Residency Training. Retrieved from <aadprt.org/training>.

HSS (U.S. Department of Health and Human Services). (2006). *Administration on children, youth and families: Child maltreatment 2004*. Washington DC: U.S. Government Printing Office.

HSS (U.S. Dept of Health and Human Services). (2010). Administration for children and families. *Mandatory reports of child abuse and neglect: Summary of state laws*. Retrieved from <www.childwelfare.gov>.

Iavicolli, L. G. (2005). Mandatory reporting of domestic violence: The law, friend or foe? *The Mount Sinai Journal of Medicine*, *72*(4), 228–231.

Levi, B. H., & Crowell, K. (2011). Child abuse experts disagree about the threshold for mandated reporting. *Clinical Pediatrics*, *50*(4), 321–329.

Locke, J. (2003). Two treatises of government. In I. Shapiro (Ed.), *Two treatises of government and a letter concerning toleration* (pp. 1–209). New Haven, CT: Yale University Press. Cited in Mathew & Bross (2008).

Mathew, B., & Bross, D. C. (2008). Mandated reporting is still a policy with reason: Empirical evidence and philosophical grounds. *Child Abuse and Neglect*, *32*, 511–516.

McManus, J., Magaret, N. D., Hedges, J. R., Rayner, N. B., & Rice, M. (2005). A survey of Oregon emergency physicians to assess mandatory reporting knowledge and reporting patterns regarding intoxicated drivers in the state of Oregon. *Academic Emergency Medicine*, *12*(9), 896–899.

Mill, J. S. (1998). On liberty. In J. Gray (Ed.), *John Stuart Mill on liberty and other essays* (pp. 5–128). Oxford, England: Oxford University Press.

Redelmeier, D. A., Vinkatesh, V., & Stanbrook, M. D. (2008). Mandatory reporting by physicians of patients potentially unfit to drive. *Open Medicine*, *2*(1), e8–e17. Epub2008 Feb 11.

Sexual Violence Justice Institute (2006). Fact sheet. Retrieved from <www.mncasa.org> via <http://bit.ly/YzEX4s>.

Shonkoff, J. P., Boyce, W. T., & McEwen, B. S. (2009). Neuroscience, molecular biology and the childhood roots of health disparities – Building a new framework for health promotion and disease prevention. Special communication. *Journal of the American Medical Association*, *301*(21), 2252–2259.

Chapter Ten

Netiquette

Etiquette is commonly associated with good manners, and good manners are part of professionalism. They convey a sense of respect towards others – our patients, our colleagues, and the entities that we work for and represent. Poor manners, whether intended or not, are subject to many different negative attributions. The health-care professional who is perceived as brusque, dismissive, rude, impatient, or unable to manage feelings appropriately risks being perceived as unprofessional. By extension, that individual's area of specialty, health-care field, institution, and profession as a whole may be cast in a negative light.

"Netiquette" is a term used for professional and polite practices online. The Internet and digital media hold all the usual potential pitfalls in terms of etiquette, as well as some pitfalls that are unique to the various digital media. Because of the speed, breadth, and permanence of digital communication, netiquette errors can quickly result in negative repercussions at the individual level for the professional who has committed the breach. But they also can lead to significant systemic impact. Who among us, for example, has not experienced an unfortunate "Reply to all" response to an email resulting in injured feelings and other negative consequences? Because of its growing importance, netiquette is being taught to young people in settings from classrooms to Girl Scout meetings; however, along with so much else that is new about technology to older generations, digital citizenship may not have been part of the education of "digital immigrants." Health-care professionals, and others, will need to learn it consciously and explicitly.

Electronic devices make netiquette breaches easier on a number of levels. The devices are small, and subject to myopic errors and keyboarding mistakes. We tend to use these devices more quickly

S. deJong: Blogs and Tweets, Texting and Friending.
DOI: http://dx.doi.org/10.1016/B978-0-12-408128-4.00010-2
© 2014 S. DeJong. Published by Elsevier Inc. All rights reserved.

than perhaps we should. The pace of digital communication leads to reflex responses without sufficient pause. Electronic communication is also limited to symbols on a screen; it lacks the nonverbal context that makes up about 90% of human communication (Mehrabian, 1972). Tone of voice, inflection, facial expression, gestures – all are missing. In their absence, even regular words can be misconstrued. The situation worsens when acronyms or abbreviations, or symbols such as emoticons, are used.

Netiquette also includes many of the issues described earlier: Concerns regarding privacy and confidentiality, and legal issues such as liability, plagiarism, and copyright. Small unintended errors in to whom a communication is sent, how content gets copied and pasted from one communication to another, or how an idea is expressed – all of these can raise significant concerns both ethically and legally.

We may use electronic devices for communicating with differing audiences in various domains of our life, from family and friends to patients, students, and colleagues. No visual cues remind us to "shift set" and adjust our communication to the audience we are addressing. Our tone, punctuation, grammar, and word choice can too easily slip into overly casual usage, and our content structure can lose a professional formality.

A critical first question before initiating any communication electronically is to decide whether that medium is the best suited to the content, remembering McLuhan's advice that "the medium is the message" (McLuhan, 1964). In health care, where safety is of paramount concern, communication in urgent situations must be carefully thought through. Using email for an urgent clinical situation, for example, is clearly not optimal (Recupero, 2009). A pervasive concern in electronic communication is that it may become an outlet for feelings that are better directed elsewhere. Use of digital media in order to vent is never appropriate.

10.1 EMAIL AND NETIQUETTE – A MODEL

In the professional world of health care, the most commonly used form of electronic communication is email, and much of what has been written about professional electronic communication relates to email. It is still a more conservative choice than either texting or social media such as tweeting. Much of what follows pertains to email but can easily be extrapolated to other forms of digital media.

Perhaps most important to remember is that electronic communication is neither private nor confidential. It is viewed by information technology personnel at institutions; by employees of software and technology hardware companies; and by the increasing array of companies whose servers are leased for the storage of information.

It is also subject to hacking and viruses, leaking, forwarding, cutting and pasting, and human error. No electronic content should be posted that the writer would not feel comfortable with other people reading. In general, sensitive or private content should not be discussed digitally. Sensitive content may be particularly subject to misinterpretation, and in general, complex feelings and ideas are not well encapsulated digitally.

Confidentiality, as discussed in Chapter 4, is a legal issue; other legal issues need to be considered as well before posting any online content. Are copyright infringements potentially involved? Are there liability concerns? Could a posting be construed as involving a conflict of interest? In addition, it may be wise to print out electronic communication and file a hard copy. For patient-related communication, this is generally required by risk management companies and others.

Other difficulties in electronic communication may fall into the ethical, if not outright legal, domain. For example, copying and pasting from one communication to another or forwarding an entire communication may constitute an ethical violation if the originator of the content is not asked for permission in advance. Similarly, "bcc-ing" recipients raises complex ethical boundary questions. If the author doesn't want the explicit recipient to know about the other recipients, is bcc the best method to use? What if an explicit recipient replies to all with sensitive content that those on the bcc list should not receive?

Other concerns fall more into the category of good manners. Respect for the recipient(s) is an important ingredient of good manners. Most health-care professionals today are overwhelmed with the amount of information they are sent on a daily basis. Email inboxes may contain thousands of emails. Thus, asking oneself whether an email is important enough to send is critical. Some people may prefer email, others may prefer other kinds of communication. Asking the intended recipient, particularly if it is someone with whom the author does not yet have a professional relationship, can prevent unintended bad feelings.

Electronic communication needs to be efficient, which means in turn it must be clear and concise. A growing body of literature catalogs how emails should be professionally constructed (Chan, 2008). Subject headings should be effective in briefly capturing the content and purpose of the email. The salutation should be appropriate to the professional context: A colleague one emails many times a day might receive an email beginning with, "Hi Dan"; however, a less familiar recipient or one who is higher up in the hierarchy may merit a "Dear Dr. So-and-so". The body of the message should reflect the content of the email. For example, Song, Halsey and Burress (2008, p. 46) recommend an "Action summary, Background and Close" format.

The action summary states in a single sentence the specific action item, purpose, or key point of the email. The background section is the body of the message that needs to be organized and structured: Group key points together using paragraphs or bullets. Be as concise and precise as possible in writing. Often, greater precision in word choice leads to greater conciseness. If attachments are included, include that in the subject heading or early on in the body. Don't send long, cumbersome attachments that will take a long time and lots of paper to print out; better to mail a hard copy. An electronic signature will authenticate the sender and also provide important information such as title and contact information.

Achieving an appropriate tone in digital communication is an art. To some extent, our goal is (to paraphrase McLuhan) to overcome the medium and assert the integrity of our message. Our professional communications should be just that – professional – but also not impersonal or distant. Errors can also engender an impersonal tone. For example, sending out a similar version of an email to multiple recipients by cutting and pasting the name in the salutation and tweaking it a little can cause Dr. Smith to receive an email that has Dr. Jones in the salutation. Careful proofreading before sending any electronic communication is vital.

Appropriate tone in digital communication can become more than a netiquette issue. Should a patient file a complaint with a state licensing board or a malpractice lawsuit, the content of any digital communication may be subject to subpoena and scrutinizing by board and jury members. Lawyers and others representing the plaintiff may seek to cast aspersions on these communications. For example, they may suggest that a tone is overly familiar in a communication between a professional and a patient (particularly if there are sexual boundary allegations involved), or raise other concerns about other implicit as well as explicit aspects of the communication.

Certain aspects of writing are best avoided in electronic communication: In general, emotionally charged language should be eschewed. All capital letters are experienced as shouting. Abbreviations and acronyms which may be second nature to the writer may be unknown, or, perhaps worse, misunderstood by the recipient. Emoticons and dramatic use of punctuation such as exclamation marks can be misconstrued and risk creating an unintended tone (for example, flippant or annoyed). Culturally limited expressions are best avoided for similar reasons. If one is dealing with a national or international audience, using terms that are accessible to all is important. Even something such as a date can be different: 01/03/2012 is January 3rd in the United States, but March

1st in Canada and Europe. Writing out the date avoids these errors. Misspellings, incorrect punctuation, and grammatical errors cast the writer in an unprofessional light, either by suggesting an inability to write correctly, or by implying that insufficient care and time has been taken to use appropriate spelling-, punctuation-, and grammar-checking software.

Sometimes we receive emails and are tempted to forward them to others out of good intent. Some examples include jokes, virus alerts, scams, hoaxes, and legends. However, forwarding incorrect information or messages that themselves include viruses is not helpful. It is best to research a message to determine its validity before sending it on.

Unfortunately, lazy responses to email lists are frequent. Rather than selecting the most appropriate recipients, senders can rely on email lists that are overly inclusive, thus cluttering inboxes and generating ill will. Similarly, sometimes responses include the entire email chain – remember to cut to only the most critical content. Finally, avoid responses that are flippant or that do not respond in a serious manner to the thread of an online conversation (Smith, 2002, p. 18).

Another important netiquette issue is response time. The capacity to respond promptly to email may depend on one's clinical setting and the various contexts in which one works. For example, in health care we may spend part of our time on hospital floors seeing patients or moving busily between examination rooms in an outpatient clinic; at other times we may be sitting at our desks. If a professional is working part-time, clear expectations need to be set with supervisors regarding response time when the professional is off-site. Response time may also differ between colleagues and administrators and patients. Different institutional cultures have different expectations in this regard; it is important to adhere to one's own cultural norms and not develop a reputation as an unreliable or slow responder. In the clinical setting, it is important to make clear with patients when they sign an informed consent (see Chapter 11) what an expected response time should be, and to emphasize that online communication should not be used for emergencies. In general, 24–72 hours is an acceptable time frame for a response (Recupero, 2009).

If you are not going to be able to respond to electronic communications within your typical time frame, perhaps because you are away or indisposed, an auto-response should be set up. The outgoing message should also be professional, providing sufficient but not excessive information and identifying who is available to help while the recipient is unavailable.

With this overview in mind, let us look at some specific examples of netiquette issues.

10.1.1 Vignettes

Consider the following vignette:

Vignette 10.1

An internist evaluates a new patient who has some neurological problems that are followed by a neurologist at a different hospital, whom the internist has heard of but does not know personally. The patient's neurological problems could be affected by the medications the internist is thinking of starting in the patient, and so there is a need to contact the neurologist to discuss possible interactions and hear about any concerns regarding the use of these medications in this patient.

Adapted from DeJong et al, 2011, Vignette #17

How should the psychiatrist contact the neurologist? Page? Email? To some extent the answer lies in the urgency of the clinical situation. If the internist does not need an immediate reply for clinical reasons, paging the neurologist seems too intrusive. However, emailing the neurologist is problematic: First, going outside of the internist's intranet system raises potential privacy issues and requires a written consent. Second, since the internist does not already have a relationship with the neurologist, email is generally not an ideal way to establish a professional relationship. If time allowed, the internist could write a letter that could document the clinical situation. Otherwise, the internist would do well to reach out by phone and find out how the neurologist would like to communicate.

Consider the content of the following vignette:

Vignette 10.2

A surgical resident receives an email announcing that two much-loved staff members on a particular service, Carol and John, are being let go as a result of budgetary cuts. The resident feels the way the institution is handling the firings is unfair and does not take into account the needs of the staff members who are longstanding employees of the hospital. She responds to the email with the following, sent after clicking "Reply to all":

This is so dumb. Can't anyone see that we are losing our best people? My heart goes out to you, Carol and John. Let me know if I can help in any way.

The resident had not noticed that the announcement was sent out on the departmental email list, and so everyone in the department, including the department chair, saw her reply.

Adapted from DeJong et al., 2011, Vignette #21

What errors of email etiquette did the resident make, and what should the resident do now? The overarching netiquette problem in this case is that the resident is using email in a reflex way to vent about strong feelings elicited by the previous email. In limbically mediated states of strong emotional arousal, our frontal lobes do not function as well; judgment and forethought are compromised. Thus, in this case, the resident does not check the distribution list on the email to notice that the department chair will be a recipient. Nor is she careful about her use of language. Words such as "dumb," especially when applied to the behavior of important administrators, are likely to generate feelings of humiliation and anger. Finally, any personal communication to recipients, such as the sentence to Carol and John, should be communicated in person offline.

Let us look now at a negative example of netiquette and then see how we might repair it:

Vignette 10.3

A medical director of an inpatient service meets with the nurse manager to share concerns that the nursing staff has not yet responded to an invitation to meet with the department chair over lunch. The director is irked by the staff's failure to respond and asks the nurse manager to make sure that the staff "gets on it." The nurse manager sends out an email to the whole nursing staff as follows:

Subject: MANDATORY LUNCH WITH CHAIR

Message: IF YOU WANT TO ATTEND LUNCH WITH THE CHAIR, RSVP TODAY, OR ELSE...

The nurses think the manager is either angry or arrogant, and decide as a group not to reply to this request, or to other requests the manager makes in subsequent weeks.

Adapted from DeJong et al., 2011, Vignette #21

This netiquette breach is an example of parallel process. The nurse manager is the victim of the medical director's anger, which is probably due to the director's own fears of looking incompetent to his chairman. In their meeting, the director projects his anger onto the nurse manager, who then attempts to offload it in the email, likely also because she does not want to look incompetent to the medical director. As a result, the nurse's email contains metaphorical shouting with the use of all caps in the subject heading, and the tone overall is dictatorial, threatening, and demeaning. Given these regressive behaviors by the nurse manager, the staff then regresses to a position of acting out on their feelings by being noncompliant. Now consider the following rewrite of the above email:

Rewrite of Vignette 10.3

Subject: RSVP to Lunch with Chair

Message: Hi all, I know you're busy, but the medical director needs to know by this Friday if you will be attending lunch with the chair next week. Please email the director's assistant as soon as you can to let her know if you can come. Thanks!

By using regular lower-case letters, neutral word choices, and a more conciliatory, polite tone, the nurse manager maintains standards of professionalism that are more likely to garner a prompt and suitable response from her staff.

Let us look beyond the content and at unprofessional behaviors around email communication. Consider this example:

Vignette 10.4

A service director receives an email from a supervisor delineating concerns about a physician's performance. The supervisor makes reference to the physician's "arrogant manner" and "tendency to dominate conversations." The service director speculates about the possible psychological origins of these alleged character traits. The service director wants to find out if other staff members are having a similar experience with the physician and forwards the supervisor's email to the service staff.

Adapted from DeJong et al., 2011, Vignette #19

Here, not only is the sensitive content inappropriate for email, but also the director takes the liberty of forwarding the email without the sender's permission. Forwarding is inappropriate because it amplifies the dissemination of sensitive content. The physician in question may well discover that the email has been disseminated, and might understandably feel "ganged up on." Rather than forwarding, the service director might talk in person and discreetly with a few key sources to learn more about the physician in question's performance.

Here is another example:

Vignette 10.5

A training director in a medical training program receives an email from a trainee complaining about a particular outpatient supervisor. The training director has been concerned about this supervisor's teaching for some time, and frustrated by a sense of impotence about how to make the situation better. The training director emails the resident back saying, "Thanks for your feedback. Let's talk about this more when you and I meet next week." Using the bcc line, the training director also sends this email to the division chief and the head of the outpatient service. The outpatient director, who has also been concerned about this supervisor, forwards the email to his friend, the inpatient medical director. Later that week, the outpatient director approaches the trainee and asks if the resident could provide some specific examples of the general complaints he had made about the supervisor in his email to the training director.

Adapted from DeJong et al., 2011, Vignette #20

This vignette exemplifies how what can feel like efficient communication via email quickly can become an inappropriate disclosure of content throughout an entire network of people, with no one person being fully aware of whom has received the information. The use of both forwarding and the "bcc" function brings people into the circle of communication unbeknownst to key people in that circle. In this case, the training director did not intend for the inpatient medical director to receive the information, nor, certainly, for the information to circle back around to the resident. Once any kind of electronic communication is sent, it becomes very difficult to control where it ends up. Thus, despite often good intent, sensitive information is inappropriately disseminated and difficult feelings are engendered: The supervisor may feel confidentiality was breached and that he was not respectfully treated; the training director may feel angry at the outpatient director for disclosing to the inpatient medical director, and so on. Obviously these boundary crossings and violations could have happened by word of mouth as well. However, the access and ease of electronic communication and its removal from the face-to-face encounter and nonverbal cues can facilitate such violations.

What is the correct response for a health-care professional who receives inappropriate information, or information that was never intended for him or her? Consider this vignette:

Vignette 10.6

A physician's assistant (PA) receives an email from the administrative coordinator at a clinical site on which the PA had worked the previous year. The email has been sent to a list of all clinicians on the site and pertains to allegations that a former supervisor on the site showed professional misconduct. This misconduct was first reported in a local newspaper, the link to which is attached. The PA is amazed and curious, and reads the attached article. He realizes that it was not intended for him since he no longer works at the site, and contacts the administrative coordinator at the clinical service to let her know that his name should be removed from the email list. He then forwards the email to colleagues on the service, and writes about his feelings regarding the news on his blog that night. He names the supervisor, saying how much he respected him and can't believe he has done something so wrong.

Adapted from DeJong et al., 2011, Vignette #22

Here, the PA very appropriately recognizes that his name was never taken off the service email list after he left the clinical site, and asks the administrator to do this. However, instead of keeping the content confidential, he proceeds to disseminate it further by emailing colleagues and blogging about the allegations regarding the supervisor. Again, we can see that emotions play a role here: The PA is upset about the allegations and needs to work through his feelings about them. However, by doing so digitally, he compromises confidentiality and propagates potential falsehood. The PA would have done better to discuss his feelings in a confidential, one-on-one conversation with a trusted colleague who is already familiar with the allegations.

Email lists and other online communities raise additional netiquette issues. Often they have their own guidelines for participation. If membership is by subscription, there are often instructions for subscribers. These guidelines and instructions should be saved for ongoing reference and adhered to. In general, they speak to concerns such as brevity and succinctness; lack of self-promotion; the importance of signing all communications and not posting anonymously; and, finally, how to unsubscribe if needed (Smith, 2002, pp. 16–17).

10.2 GENERAL RECOMMENDATIONS FOR PROPER NETIQUETTE

Digital media, like all media, have their own characteristics and limitations. Health-care professionals should choose the best medium for a specific task. They should try to separate professional from personal communication portals; if this is not possible, they should pause when shifting between different contexts and audiences. Recall that electronic communication is not private unless specifically protected by encryption and other security measures.

Professional protocol requires particular attention to word choice, tone, grammar, and punctuation. Communications should be organized, brief but complete, and sent only to those who need to receive them. Authentication methods such as electronic signature and documents of authentication assure recipients that the email is from you. Cutting and pasting, forwarding, bcc-ing, and replying to all can be appropriate at times, but should be carefully considered prior to acting.

The frame around the use of electronic communication needs to be set up ahead of time: What purpose each medium will be used for; what the expected response time will be; the best way to reach the professional in an emergency, and so on. If there is a shift in frame, for example the professional is out of the office, that change needs to be clearly indicated with an "out-of-office" reply.

CONCLUSION

Good manners online are not a trivial matter. They reflect the individual's professionalism as well as the professionalism of the institution and field that the practitioner represents. Because of the unique characteristics of digital communication, including the speed, scope, permanence, and lack of nonverbal cues, it lends itself to netiquette errors. Health-care professionals would do well to learn how to use digital media such as email professionally and effectively in order to present themselves, their institutions, and their field in the most positive light possible.

REFERENCES

Chan, J.F. (2008). E-mail – A write it well guide. How to write and manage e-mail in the workplace. Oakland, CA: <Writeitwell.com>.

DeJong, S. M., Benjamin, S., Anzia, J. M., John, N., Boland, R. J., Lomax, J., et al. (2011). Curriculum on professionalism and the Internet in psychiatry. *Academic Psychiatry*, *36*(5), 356–362. http://dx.doi.org/doi:10.1176. Retrieved from <aadprt.org>.

McLuhan, M. (1964). Understanding media: The extensions of man. New York: Mentor; reissued in 1994 Cambridge, MA: MIT Press.

Mehrabian, A. U. (1972). *Nonverbal communication*. Oxford, England: Aldine-Atherton.

Recupero, P. R. (2009). Email and the psychiatrist–patient relationship. *Journal of the American Academy of Psychiatry and the Law*, *33*, 465–467.

Smith, L.A. (2002) Business e-Mail – How to make it professional and effective. San Anselmo CA: Writing and Editing at Work. <Writingandeditingatwork.com>.

Song, M., Halsey, V., & Burress, T. (2008). *The hamster revolution*. San Francisco, CA: Berrett-Koehler.

Chapter Eleven

Recommendations for Professional Use of Social Media, Digital Technology, and the Internet

If the preceding chapters have been convincing that maintaining professional behavior online is vital for all health-care professionals, then the next question is how does the health-care professional achieve this goal? As Chapter 12 will discuss, the major challenge is that technology and its interface with health care is a moving target: Technological innovations seem to occur daily, and we are undergoing a paradigm shift in terms of the ways in which patients and health-care professionals relate to technology and integrate it into their routine practice. For this reason, detailed recommendations that have long-lasting value are virtually impossible since they will so quickly become obsolete. This chapter, therefore, will focus on broader concepts, starting with general recommendations about Internet use and moving on to recommendations specific to many of the current forms of digital media. Suggestions are offered with the caveat that some aspects of even these recommendations could soon be out of date. One additional disclaimer: I am not a lawyer and in no way are these recommendations intended as legal advice or advice about how to handle a particular situation, especially one with a patient. They are a place to start. All health-care professionals

S. deJong: Blogs and Tweets, Texting and Friending.
DOI: http://dx.doi.org/10.1016/B978-0-12-408128-4.00011-4
© 2014 S. DeJong. Published by Elsevier Inc. All rights reserved.

should be aware of the standards about technology where they practice, and obtain appropriate consultation as necessary.

First, and perhaps most important, health-care professionals should use the most appropriate means of communication for a given task, not forgetting that sometimes the most appropriate means is a face-to-face conversation. When content is sensitive or has the potential to elicit difficult feelings, face-to-face contact almost always ensures better communication by including nonverbal aspects. If the relationship between the sender and recipient is already delicate, or if a power differential exists, particular care needs to be taken. When a face-to-face interaction is impossible, telephone is probably the next best choice.

Next, professionals using technology need to know how to use it responsibly, safely, and effectively. For "digital immigrants," achieving comfort with the ever-growing array of technology can be a major challenge. If they find it difficult, the most prudent course is to proceed gradually and not take on more than can be managed. For some digital immigrants, telephone voicemails and emails may be as much as they can handle administratively. Even for digital natives, who according to the Pew data are the ones most likely to start using the newest technologies as soon as they become available, the risk of having multiple communication pathways to maintain and respond to can be daunting (Jones, 2009; Zickuhr, 2012). Technology users need to understand the limitations and issues inherent in technological communication, such as: lack of confidentiality and privacy; permanence; liability to rapid dissemination without the author's knowledge, including forwarding and cutting and pasting; the ways in which any data placed online can be aggregated and used to form impressions about someone that will be used by businesses and potentially others; and other key issues discussed in preceding chapters.

At a more technological level, people need to understand how to use the technology so as to minimize concerns in these areas; for example, how to use privacy settings and know when they are reset by the software owner; how to encrypt content if necessary; how to provide electronic signatures and use other authentication tools; how to block outgoing content like cell-phone numbers; how to password-protect all devices (desktop and mobile), and so on. Developing a strong, ongoing work relationship with the IT department where one works can be key.

Increasingly, health-care institutions, licensing boards, medical schools, professional associations, and malpractice insurance providers are providing guidelines for appropriate use of digital media (Box 11.1). No single, complete, uniform standard has yet emerged; and such a standard may prove impossible given the constant flux in

BOX 11.1   Existing Guidelines and Sample Policies

- American Academy of Orthopaedic Surgeons (2012). Social media in healthcare – A primer for orthopaedic surgeons. Retrieved from http://www3.aaos.org/member/prac_manag/Social_Media_Healthcare_Primer.pdf
- American Association of Directors of Psychiatry Residency Training (2011). Curriculum on professionalism and the Internet. Retrieved from http://bit.ly/Y42Jus
- American Medical Association (2010). Professionalism in the use of social media. http://bit.ly/zpSrXf
- American Psychiatric Association (2009). The Internet in clinical psychiatry (resource document), Joint Reference Committee. Retrieved from http://www.psychiatry.org
- American Psychological Association (1997). APA Statement on services by telephone, teleconferencing and internet. A statement by the Ethics Committee of the APA
- Australian Medical Association (2011). Social media and the medical profession – A guide to online professionalism for medical practitioners and medical students. Retrieved from https://ama.com.au/social-media-and-medical-profession
- British Medical Association (2012). Social media use: Practice and ethical guidance for doctors and medical students. Obtainable from: http://bma.org.uk/practical-support-at-work/ethics/ethics-a-to-z
- Clinical Social Work Federation (2001). CSWF Position paper on internet text-based therapy. http://bit.ly/ZqCxde
- eRisk Working Group for Healthcare (2002). Guidelines for online communication. http://www.medem.com/phy/phy_eriskguidelines.cfm
- Faust R. Developing a social media policy for your hospital practice. Retrieved from http://bit.ly/rapdZl
- Federation of State Medical Boards, Inc. (2002). Model guidelines for the appropriate use of the internet in medical practice. Retrieved from http://www.fsmb.org/pdf/2002_grpol_use_of_internet.pdf
- Federation of State Medical Boards, Inc. (2012). Model policy guidelines for the appropriate use of social media and social networking in medical practice. Retrieved from www.fsmb.org/pdf/pub-social-media-guidelines.pdf
- Health on the Net Foundation (1996). Principles. Retrieved from http://www.hon.ch/HONcode/Conduct.html
- Healthcare bloggers code of ethics. Downloaded from http://medbloggercode.com/the-code/
- Hi-Ethics (2000). Health Internet ethics: Ethical principles for offering internet health services to consumers. Retrieved from http://www.hiethics.com/Principles/index.asp
- Hsiung, R. (2002). Suggested principles of professional ethics for e-therapy. In R. Hsiung (Ed.) e-therapy: Case studies, guiding principles and the clinical potential of the internet. New York, NY: WW. Norton, pp. 150–165
- Interdisciplinary telehealth standards working group (1999). Core principles on telehealth, Washington, DC: American Nursing Publishing
- International Society for Mental health online and psychiatric society for informatics (2000). The suggested principles for the online provision of mental health services. Retrieved from http://www.ismho.org
- Massachusetts Medical Society (2012). Social media guidelines for physicians. Retrieved from http://www.massmed.org/socialmedia

- Ohio State University Medical Center (2009). Social media participation guidelines. Downloaded from http://bit.ly/dcrvr6
- National Board for Certified Counselors and Center for Credentialing and Education (2001). The practice of internet counseling. Retrieved from http://www.nbcc.org/ethics/webethics.htm
- National Council of State Boards of Nursing. White Paper: A nurse's guide to the use of social media. Retrieved from http://www.ncsbn.org/11_NCSBN_Nurses_Guide_Social_Media.pdf
- US Department of Health and Human Services (1996). Health Insurance Portability and Accountability Act. Retrieved from http://www.hhs.gov/ocr/privacy
- Vanderbilt University Medical Center. VUMC Social media policy. Retrieved from http://bit.ly/bqLlqS

technology and its use in our society. It is up to individual health-care professionals to be familiar with the policies, standards, and requirements of their institutions, boards, professional associations, and malpractice insurers, as well as health-care laws such as the Health Insurance Portability and Accountability Act (HIPAA). Adhering to these standards is important not only for one's current employment but also for any future employment or training opportunity, as potential employers and training programs are increasingly searching for online content about applicants before making a decision about them.

Set the frame ahead of time. Too often, practitioners get into trouble with technology because they have headed down a slippery slope without anticipating and thinking through potential repercussions. Having a "Notice of privacy practices" to distribute to patients that clearly outlines routine use of technology is vital and legally required in many circumstances. In addition, written informed consent about specific use of media needs to be signed by patient and provider, and can be tailored to the individual circumstances of the patient (for example, use of an informed consent for email and texts in a situation where a multidisciplinary care team is involved and communication is vital). Privacy policies, informed consent, and the allied documentation need to be revisited frequently as a way for providers to remind patients of continuing concerns around their use of technology.

With the increasing use of mobile devices for email and other functions (an estimated 80% of physicians use a mobile device on the job), health-care professionals need to know how to protect their mobile devices from confidentiality breaches. An experiment by Symantec in which 50 smartphones were "lost" in five different cities, and then the finders of the phones followed up, discovered that half of the time, finders tried to return the phone, but 96% of them also looked at the data stored on the phone (Dolan, 2012).

For hospitals and larger practices, hiring a professional security firm to secure mobile devices may make sense. For small practices and individual providers, efforts might include the following recommendations adapted from Dolan (2012):

1. Buy the right device (explain the sensitivity of the information and your encryption needs to the vendor);
2. Use a high-quality encryption app;
3. Use a passcode to access the device; some of these passcodes can automatically wipe the device after a number of failed login attempts;
4. Have the capacity to wipe the device remotely if it is lost (recognizing that all data, not just sensitive data, will be lost);
5. Add another layer between the main menu of the phone and access to confidential content.

As is so often the case in health care, when a practitioner has doubts or questions about how to proceed with technology, obtaining consultation is essential. Depending on the nature of the uncertainty, a practitioner might contact a hospital administrator, IT specialist, a legal expert, an ethics expert, or a clinical consultant. As with all consultations that pertain to a specific patient, the nature of and recommendations from the consultation should be documented in the medical record.

Finally, for any digitally generated content, care should be taken not to violate the important professionalism standards raised in this book: standard of care and liability concerns (including unlicensed practice, boundary issues, and inadvertently creating a treatment relationship); patient confidentiality and security of patient information; patient and practitioner privacy; libel; conflict of interest; issues of academic integrity; safety and mandated reporting requirements; and netiquette. As the Federation of State Medical Boards (FSMB, 2002, p. 2) comments:

> *The appropriate application of … technology can enhance medical care by facilitating communication with physicians and other health care providers, refilling prescriptions, obtaining laboratory results, scheduling appointments, monitoring chronic conditions, providing health care information and clarifying medical advice. However, it is the expectation of the Board that e-mail and other electronic communications and interactions between the physician and patient should supplement and enhance, but not replace, crucial interpersonal interactions that create the very basis of the physician-patient relationship.*

The FSMB specifically states that it is the Board's expectation that physicians providing medical care, whether electronically or otherwise, "maintain a high degree of professionalism and should: place the welfare of the patient first; maintain acceptable standards of practice; adhere to recognized ethical codes governing the medical profession; properly supervise physician extenders; [and] protect patient confidentiality" (FSMB, 2002, p. 2).

Let us now turn to professional use of different kinds of digital media. We will discuss email, blogs and professional websites, texts, search engines, and social media and media-sharing sites.

11.1 EMAIL

In 2012, The Cochrane Collaboration published a meta-analysis reviewing nine published studies (1,733 patients) on the use of email between health-care professionals and patients, with the goal of providing recommendations for use of email in clinical practice (Atherton, Sawmynaden, Sheikh, Majeed & Car, 2012). The authors attempted to examine seven outcome measures: patient's understanding, patient health status and wellbeing, patient/caregiver views, patient behaviors and action, health service outcome/resource use, health professional outcomes, and harms. The quality of the evidence was deemed to be "very low" in the first five of those categories, and unable to be measured in the latter two. The authors concluded: "The nature of the results means that we cannot make any recommendations for how email might best be used in clinical practice" (Atherton, Sawmynaden, Sheikh, Majeed & Car, 2012, p. 2). (Given this dearth of data on appropriate use of email, which has been available since the 1990s in most health-care settings, one might imagine how little data exists about other technologies.)

Some codes of ethics, such as those of the American Psychological Association, address these issues, although compliance with these guidelines has been shown to be low (American Psychological Association, 1997; Maheu & Gordon, 2000; Welfel & Bunce, 2003). However, because email has been in use for longer than other digital technologies, some guidelines do exist. In 2000, the American Medical Association (AMA) published guidelines based on the work of Beverly Kane and Daniel Sands, which grew out of a taskforce of the American Medical Informatics Association (American Medical Association, 1999; Kane & Sands, 1998). Importantly, these and other guidelines generally pertain to situations in which "the health care provider has taken on an explicit measure of responsibility for the client's care." They do not apply to unsolicited emails or situations in which "no contractual relationship exists, as in an online discussion group in a public support forum" (Kane & Sands, 1998, p. 104). Eysenbach (2000, p. 19) distinguishes between "Type A encounters," i.e. those that occur in the absence of a pre-existing relationship, and "Type B encounters," in which a bona fide relationship, either through traditional clinical care or telemedicine, already exists. These latter situations raise the difficult legal question of whether a doctor–patient relationship has been established. Even the FSMB acknowledges that it may be difficult in some circumstances, particularly in an online setting, to define precisely the beginning of the physician–patient relationship.

> *[It] tends to begin when an individual seeks assistance from a physician with a health-related matter for which the physician may provide assistance. However, the relationship is clearly established when the physician agrees to undertake diagnosis and treatment of the patient and the patient agrees, whether or not there has been a personal encounter between the physician (or other supervised health care practitioner) and patient.*

FSMB, 2002, p. 4

The FSMB also stipulates that the initiation of such a relationship should take the form of a face-to-face evaluation and examination (p. 5).

It is also important to distinguish between email used in the business of ongoing clinical care (making appointments, requesting prescription refills) and "e-therapy" (a term particularly used in the mental health field; Hsiung, 2002) or "e-health," a term referring to health-care practice facilitated by electronic communication. In both e-therapy and e-health, email may be a vehicle for providing actual care to the patient. The following recommendations pertain to situations in which email is being used for administrative purposes and also for the provision of care with the explicit agreement of both provider and patient, i.e. not in situations of unsolicited email or no contractual agreement to provide care. These latter situations will be addressed at the end of this section.

11.1.1 Use of Email with Informed Consent

First, reasonable measures to protect the confidentiality of email communication with patients (and with others involved in the patient's care) should be taken (Kane & Sands, 1998, pp. 106–107; Recupero, 2005, p. 467). Encryption is a method by which a sender can transform readable text into an unintelligible message which can then be decrypted by the recipient, typically using a password. According to the American Bar Association, encrypted email "affords a reasonable expectation of privacy from a technological and legal standpoint" (American Bar Association, 1999, cited in Recupero, 2005 p. 467). The use of protected portals by medical practices and institutions also offers protection against confidentiality breaches. As Recupero points out: "The chance of misdirection and interception on this secure network is substantially less than in the case of e-mail accounts hosted by Internet service providers." Firewalls, electronic signature and authentication methods, and confirmation of receipt all enhance the protection of email content (Recupero, 2005, p. 468).

An important emerging standard is the use of written informed consent for the use of email with patients. The FSMB (2002) requires a written agreement to be in place, which has been discussed with the patient and then signed by them. This agreement is then placed in the medical record. According to the FSMB, it should include the following terms:

- *Types of transmissions that will be permitted (prescription refills, appointment scheduling, patient education, etc.)*
- *Under what circumstances alternate forms of communication or office visits should be utilized*
- *Security measures: such as encrypting data, password, protected screen savers and data files, or utilizing other reliable authentication techniques, as well as potential risks to privacy*
- *Hold-harmless clause for information lost due to technical failures*
- *Requirement for express patient consent to forward patient-identifiable information to a third party*
- *Patient's failure to comply with the agreement may result in physician terminating the email relationship.*

FSMB, 2002, p. 6

Thus, an email consent form can be used to outline the potential risks and benefits of using email and the responsibilities for both patient and practitioner when it is used. It should include delineation of confidentiality (who will have access to emails, whether they will be in the chart, to whom they may be forwarded); expected turnaround time; when not to use email (such as when content is too sensitive or the situation emergent); and how to use subject headings effectively. Some providers may want to use the consent as a waiver for encryption. Informed consent is a process, not a form; the signing of the consent form should be accompanied by a discussion of its content and this content will need to be reviewed in an ongoing way with the patient (Recupero, 2005, p. 468).

Additional information on the consent might pertain to financial issues such as whether the health-care provider will bill for time answering emails. Indemnification of the provider for technical failure that results in failure of transmission is also important.

Technical failures might include viruses, incorrect email address (as long as due diligence has been paid to obtaining a correct one), failure of software, power outages, and so on. Finally, the patient's and the provider's right to revoke the email consent and the practice of using email provides important safeguards in cases in which patients change their mind or providers have concerns that the modality is not suitable for use with a particular patient.

In general, experts advise that email communication be downloaded into the chart with patient identifiers (e.g. name and date of birth). Of course, if this is the standard, then failure to download emails may open the provider up to liability concerns. However, having emails in the chart is often essential for ongoing documentation of care.

The FSMB also recommends having an automatic reply to email that acknowledges messages have been delivered and read. It also suggests that "patients should be encouraged to confirm that they have received and read messages" (FSMB, 2002, p. 5). Stating in the automatic reply that email is not an appropriate method for communicating in emergencies, and providing emergency contact information, may also be appropriate.

As discussed in Chapter 10, tone, word choice, punctuation, and spelling all need to be professional. Emails should be brief and straightforward. If the email starts to become lengthy, it may be a sign that a different form of communication, such as a phone call or a mailed or faxed report, would be preferable. Similarly, if the provider becomes aware of writing hurriedly, sloppily, or with lots of feeling, then he or she may need to pause before sending the email. One option is to draft the email and then wait before sending it (the "24-hour rule"); the provider, on further reflection, may realize that a personal conversation is a better way to communicate.

Practitioners should beware of using email in a way that might constitute practicing care across state lines if the practitioner is not licensed in the state in which the patient is currently located. This issue is less concerning for the patient who travels occasionally, but most concerning for the student who goes away to school or the patient who moves but wants to continue care. If the practitioner feels it is important to provide care to the patient in this setting, it may be advisable to contact the state medical board in the other state to determine what that state's requirements are in this regard.

11.1.2 Unsolicited Emails

Let us now turn to the question of unsolicited emails. The crux of this issue is well put by Eysenbach, who led the international Internet Healthcare Coalition (IHC) which organized an e-Health ethics summit in Washington, DC in the winter of 2000. Dr. Eysenbach wrote: "Patients have to be educated that it is unethical to diagnose and treat over the Internet in the absence of a pre-existing patient–physician relationship, even if the interaction is limited to a single email" (Eysenbach, 2000, p. 2). It is necessary to determine, as discussed in Chapter 3, what constitutes a patient–physician relationship and what constitutes providing patient care (recall Blum's four categorizations of online medical activity). Standards are different internationally. For example, the German professional code states that "no physician may give individual medical treatment, including medical advice, neither exclusively by mail… nor exclusively over communication media or computer communication networks" (Eysenbach, 2000, p. 9). On the other hand, the British General Medical Council in a note on "Providing advice and medical service on-line or by telephone" does not prohibit use of email advice, leaving the question to the discretion and judgment of the individual physician. What does seem clear is that, "the more health information is personalized and tailored to the individual, and the more it encourages the receiver to act upon the advice, the more we are moving within the continuum from giving general health advice towards attempting to treat, and therefore practicing medicine" (p. 7).

Some have argued that unsolicited emails should simply be deleted, citing the "first do no harm" principle of ethics (Huntley, 1999). Risk management and legal advisors tend to offer conservative advice, noting that in this large gray zone, a cautious approach is the best way to avoid trouble (Vanderpool, 2012). Eysenbach and others argue that, despite the limitations of electronic communication, we also have an ethical obligation to educate patients and consumers. Not responding is not only unethical but also disrespectful, rude, and "a slap in the face to those who argue that patients should be informed, educated, and encouraged to take responsibility for their own health. Already, patients are largely turning to the Internet because they think that physicians do not take enough time for their concerns" (Reents & Miller, 1998).

Rather than click Delete, health-care professionals, according to Eysenbach, should read the email and help the sender find someone who can help them. With the sender's permission, the email may be forwarded. A clearance center for unsolicited emails is one suggestion. If a professional has a website with an email address associated with it, a standard reply might be in order. Such a reply could include other sources of information.

Some practitioners have relied on the use of disclaimers, including automatic replies that state that emails are not a proper way to initiate a professional–patient relationship. While not illegal, such disclaimers have not been found to be reliable in court, and the AMA has stated that disclaimers do not provide absolution from the ethical responsibility to attend to patients' interests (Eysenbach, 2002, p. 8; Recupero, 2005, p. 470).

What should a health-care professional do in face of an unsolicited email? Eysenbach offers six suggested principles for giving Type A teleadvice on the Internet:

1. *Physicians responding to patients' requests on the Internet should act within the limitations of telecommunication services and keep the global nature of the Internet in mind.*
2. *Not every aspect of medicine requires face-to-face communication or physical examination, thus teleadvice may be legitimate in some cases.*
3. *Requests for help, including unsolicited patient questions, should not be ignored, but dealt with in some manner.*
4. *Informed consent requires fair and honest labeling (disclaimers and disclosures).*
5. *Health professionals and information providers must maintain confidentiality.*
6. *Health professionals should define internal procedures and perform quality control measures.*

Eysenbach, 2002, p. 12

In Principle 1, Eysenbach includes a list of "don'ts:" don't make specific diagnoses (emphasize that any diagnoses can only be made by a treating physician); don't prescribe medicines; don't provide advice around or challenge the advice/treatment provided by other professionals without knowing the case well; don't make comments about general information that looks like individualized information; don't make your suspected diagnoses explicit (e.g. don't say something could be cancer); don't give detailed advice if you don't know the sender's ethnic, national or cultural background.

Regarding Principle 2, Eysenbach specifically mentions drug information and preventive medicine (lifestyle counseling, nutrition, primary and tertiary prevention). He recommends the following:

- *Encourage the patient to see a doctor if you feel the patient should, and if the patient seems to be reluctant for some irrational reason.*
- *Provide addresses of self-support groups and other organizations which may provide help and support.*
- *Provide addresses of specialists and hospitals.*
- *Answer general questions on side effects of medicines.*

- *Answer general questions on the compatibility of certain drugs and identify combinations of drugs which may pose problems.*
- *Give your opinion on whether certain symptoms should be investigated.*
- *Answer questions on prevention of diseases and injuries.*
- *Recommend simple measures which may alleviate the problem.*
- *Try to identify questions the patient should ask himself to decide whether or not to see a doctor.*
- *Provide emotional support.*
- *Provide general information, e.g. disease fact sheets, the latest research results and information on ongoing trials; but make it clear that this is general information which may not apply to the patient's individual case and should be discussed with the treating physician.*
- *Refer to areas of uncertainties.*

Eysenbach, 2002

The remaining principles pertain to the notion that the email sender has a right to know how emails will be stored and handled and what the risks of email are. In addition, the qualification of the responder and any potential conflicts of interest need to be disclosed. Ideally, health-care institutions should have a system for triaging unsolicited emails. Finally, every effort needs to be made to encourage the patient to obtain face-to-face medical evaluation, when appropriate.

In conclusion, while experts disagree on how to respond appropriately to unsolicited emails and professionals are urged to comply with the requirements of their practice and jurisdiction, it may be reasonable to respond in a manner that is helpful without providing such individually tailored or specific advice that it could be construed as initiating a patient–provider relationship and practicing medical care.

11.2 PROFESSIONAL WEBSITES, BLOGS, AND CHAT ROOMS

Professional blogs and websites which provide health-care information, as well as the less formal chat rooms, often fall into Eysenbach's category of Type A encounters in which patient and health-care provider have no pre-existing relationship; the provider is not explicitly assuming responsibility for the patient; contact is typically initiated by the patient; and information about the patient's circumstances is typically limited to what the patient provides through electronic text or, potentially, photographs (Eysenbach, 2002, p. 19). Thus, the six principles discussed above under "unsolicited emails" apply equally in these cases.

For blogging specifically, the Healthcare Bloggers Code of Ethics provides five standards for health and wellness blogs (http://www .medbloggercode.com/the-code/):

1. **Clear representation of perspective** – This standard suggests that readers have the right to know about authors' perspectives and expertise. It includes distinguishing between advertisement and content. Although it does not preclude anonymous blogging, in general anonymity is coming under increasing disfavor.
2. **Confidentiality** – This standard emphasizes the need for HIPAA compliance.
3. **Commercial disclosure** – This standard requires disclosure of any potential conflicts of interest pertaining to commerce. (I would add that any potential conflict of interest should be disclosed since it informs how the reader interprets the content.)
4. **Reliability of information** – Sources need to be cited and any errors corrected or pointed out.
5. **Courtesy** – This standard prohibits personal attacks, emphasizing that blogs are a forum for discussion of the merits of ideas not the people who espouse them.

To these I would add:

6. **Exercise restraint** when posting content, especially personal and patient content. Beware of humor, shop talk, and criticism. Remember it is our job to maintain appropriate boundaries and present ourselves, our specialties, the health-care profession, and any institutions we are affiliated with in a professional manner.
7. **Do not vent** online.
8. If you discuss general medical advice, make it clear that you are not in a treatment relationship with any individual online.
9. Remember that you are responsible for all content on your blog or website.

11.3 TEXTS

B.J. Fogg, the Director of the Stanford Persuasive Technology Laboratory, who authored a book entitled *Mobile Persuasion: 20 Perspectives on the Future of Behavior Change* (Fogg & Eckles, 2007), studies how technology and, especially, mobile platforms can be used to change peoples' attitudes and behaviors. At a conference on Texting4Health that Fogg organized, a representative from the National Center for Health Marketing at the Center for Disease Control (CDC), Janice R. Nall, presented the topic "Why CDC cares about Mobile Health." She cited 12 attributes of texting:

1. Always on and with you [consider how mobile phyisicians are]
2. Reaches across demographic lines – underserved populations, younger generations, etc. (Hoffman, 2012)

3. Contextual
4. Inexpensive to own
5. Two-way communications – engagement opportunities
6. Emergency alerting tool
7. Surveillance tool – not just dissemination or engagement
8. Immediacy of action and response
9. Measurable results
10. Portability
11. Geographical positioning
12. Text, audio, and video.

Not surprising, then, texting is one of the new frontiers of e-health. (See Chapter 12 for more applications of texting in the future.) To date, most use with patients has focused on compliance issues such as appointment reminders (see discussion of Intelecare Compliance Solutions Inc., New Haven CT and Smile Reminder, Lehi, UT in Terry, 2008). A recent study conducted in four London, England, mental health clinics found that texting patients appointment reminders reduced the no-show rate (Sims et al., 2012). Physician-based text messaging focuses on providing medical information to providers through their smartphones. For example, DocAlerts, a free service of Epocrates, Inc., sends more than 2 million messages per month to their users providing information specific to their area of clinical practice. The alert is linked to further information and resources, and how users respond also informs Epocrates about the content areas about which providers are seeking information.

The same features that make texting so appealing to the CDC's Center for Health Marketing, as well as some additional features, make it problematic from a professionalism standpoint. The confidentiality and security of the information is an important obstacle. A growing number of private entities are offering HIPAA-compliant texting technologies that are encrypted and in some cases download directly to the medical record (see, for example, mHealthText; www.mobilehealthrx.com). However, these do not address issues such as ensuring that correct phone numbers are dialed, knowing that the intended recipient answers the phone and that the particular phone encrypts content, or controlling the content of the patient's response (remembering that providers, not patients, are obligated under the HIPAA Privacy Rule (available at www.hhs.gov).

Other limitations of texting include character limits. Texts include SMS (short message service) and other technologies that include ANSI CDMA networks, Digital AMPS, satellite and landline networks, and multimedia messaging service (MMS), which includes images, audio, video, and rich text (Terry, 2008,

p. 520). Because they generally have a 140-character limitation, text-writers often seek to cut corners by limiting words and using unique texting vocabulary. The latter can be easily misunderstood; for example "ty" means "thank you;" "brb" means "be right back;" and "imo" means "in my opinion." New vocabulary is being developed all the time (p. 522).

The American Telemedicine Association (ATA), which has issued practice guidelines in other areas of telemedicine, has discussed guidelines on use of texting. However, the ATA website currently offers no such guidelines (http://www.americantelemed.org).

Online blogs remain a useful source of information on this issue. The following guidelines, adapted from Ericka L. Adler's blog on the Physicians Practice website, may prove useful (Adler, 2012):

1. Don't use your personal phone number to text from unless you intend to use it for patient access (which I do not recommend). Use a computer or a service that de-identifies the sender's number, or use a separate mobile device for personal and professional applications. (Some technologies such as GoogleVoice provide a way to do this on a single device).

2. Having a patient's cell phone number does not constitute permission to text the patient. Like email use with patients, texting requires a specific consent process and form delineating the risks and benefits and how it will be used in each case.

3. The Federal Communications Commission (FCC) sets certain standards regarding texting. For example messages cannot be sent to wireless phones via an auto-dialer. Practitioners should review their texting practices with legal counsel.

4. Be aware of what fees are incurred by patients for text messages you send them. If your practice will charge an additional fee, for example for appointment reminders, this needs to be made explicit in the informed consent and written agreement provided by the patient.

5. Update patients' phone numbers regularly. A text sent to a third party instead of the patient, even if inadvertently, can pose the risk of a privacy violation.

6. Optimize the security of text messages, for example by using encryption or other secure technologies typically involving password-protection. Delineate the security efforts and limitations in the written informed consent.

7. Save texts in the patient record if they constitute medical decision-making about a patient. Even if they don't, certain licensing boards have requirements around how long communications with patients need to be kept; providers should know the applicable regulations in their jurisdiction.

11.4 SEARCH ENGINES

The use of search engines in health-care practice encompasses two broad areas: our patients searching for or inadvertently finding information about us, and we health-care professionals searching for or inadvertently finding information about our patients. These will be addressed in turn.

11.4.1 Protecting the Provider

Providers need to know what content is available about them on the Internet (Mostaghimi, Crotty, & Landono, 2010). Such knowledge is best achieved by regular online searches on one's own name. However, Internet users should be aware that we live in what has been termed a "surveillance economy," and much is known about us through our use of the Internet by people we are completely unaware of (Singer, 2012): In the face of growing demand regarding personal habits, online activities, and information about consumers, personal data is collected systematically all the time, both online and offline. This information is then sold to a range of users, including marketing firms, technology companies, and government agencies. All of us have left not just a foot print but a trail of information about ourselves through our smartphone use, online shopping, and postings on blogs and social media sites (Farrell, 2012). Many websites place small files, cookies, on a computer after the user visits a website, and these then track the user's online activity. This information is then collected by data brokers (sometimes known as information resellers), stored, and sold to "financial services firms, insurance companies, law enforcement agencies, attorneys, and others" (Farrell, 2012, p. B5).

By combining this information with offline data such as legal records, detailed profiles about people can be constructed. Privacy firms have discovered that erasing negative content from online sources is difficult and so they focus instead on making their clients less "visible" (Farrell, 2012, p. B7). The Federal Trade Commission is pushing for greater transparency regarding how online companies and data brokers collect data; however, at the time of writing, no regulations exist in this regard.

Nonetheless, the best method of protecting one's online identity remains ongoing vigilance. Broad search engines such as Google, Bing, and Yahoo are typically a good place to start, since they are what patients seem most likely to use to look up their health-care providers. Don't forget old online accounts and dating sites where your personal information may still be available. Using quotation marks around one's name makes the search more efficient. For example, "John Q. Smith" will provide a list of all references to this full name instead of all the mentions of "John" and "Smith," which will be numerous. Sites such as spokeo.com will show users a picture of their home and, for a fee, even more information can be obtained. Using aggregate blog searchers such as blogsearch.google.com or blog-searchengine.com can be an efficient method. In addition, online services exist that will alert subscribers to mention of their name online.

Consider using the services of a professional online privacy firm. Companies such as Abine Inc., PrivacyChoice, and Reputation.com Inc. provide services to help people control personal information about them on the Web. These services are not free. They can be more effective at helping protect one's online reputation going forward than removing past content, for example, Abine sends a report every 3 months outlining what they have found about you online (Richmond, 2011, p. 2).

If a health-care provider discovers unflattering content about him- or herself online, the best first approach is to contact the website owner or manager in an effort to remove the embarrassing or incorrect content. Many data brokers will allow consumers to opt out of their databases (Richmond, 2011, pp. 2–3). Information that is taken down from a particular website should disappear off a Google search within weeks.

Online rating sites, which have become increasingly common, pose particular problems. In 2012, over 80 doctor rating sites existed according to Jeffrey Segal (Segal, 2012), and they have an aggregate effect. Often they are anonymous, so the source of the information (potentially a disgruntled patient or an imposter) is not known. The postings are rarely representative of an entire practice. A couple of bad ratings may actually be perceived as creating an overall more credible picture than uniformly good ones (Segal, 2012, p. 342). Inappropriate rating content (for example, those containing abusive or inflammatory language) may constitute a violation of the Terms of Use policy of the site; however, negative comments may reflect legitimate dissatisfaction with services provided. Segal cites an example of a dentist successfully reaching out to a dissatisfied patient offline after reading the patient's negative online rating. Online responses are not encouraged due to privacy and HIPAA concerns.

One study suggests that most online reviews of physicians are favorable (Tehrani, Feldman, Camacho, & Balkirshnan, 2011). Thus, encouraging patients to share a positive experience may be a way to put any negative content in a broader, more realistic context. eMerit is a firm offering assistance by uploading positive survey data. However, this approach, which is advocated by Segal and an organization called Medical Justice, can easily backfire, as is evidenced by a class action alleging that a New York dentist attempted to use online copyright law to gag patients' online reviews of her services (Lee, 2011). The plaintiffs apparently alleged that the dentist required them to sign a "Mutual agreement to maintain privacy." Practitioners should avoid all coercive practices. They should also be familiar with the Federal Trade Commission's "Guides concerning the use of endorsements and testimonials in advertising."

Lawsuits for defamation and libel are an option but not a promising one. One exception occurred in Arizona in 2011 in which a jury awarded a $12 million judgment to two doctors after a local jazz singer criticized their practice on Internet reviews and filed complaints with the state Medical Board (Alltucker, 2011). In general, however, it appears difficult to prove that online comments do not constitute opinion, which is not subject to defamation laws. And a lawsuit, particularly with significant media coverage, might amplify rather than conceal the negative allegations.

By far the best way to minimize the effect of negative content about oneself online is to generate positive content. Having a professional website and other web pages that will rise to the top of search engine results is a way of generating such content. Any "skeletons" that exist will drop down lower and may require downward scrolling and clicking to subsequent screens to find. Judicious use of links to reputable sites can also affect in what order one's data emerges on an online search result. (In linking to other sites, care should be taken that they are of high quality and no conflict of interest exists with the existing site; such a conflict should be disclosed.) Ensuring that positive content will be elicited by knowing what kinds of keywords are typically entered on searches can also be helpful.

11.4.2 Protecting the Patient

As we have discussed, online information is in the public domain. Technically speaking, therefore, we health-care providers have a right to obtain online information about our patients. Nonetheless, as Clinton, Silverman, & Brendel (2010) so clearly elucidate in their article on patient-targeted googling, before performing an online search of a patient, providers would do well to ask themselves six questions (see Box 5.1).

The question "Why do I want to conduct this search?" is seminal and requires honest introspection. Providers must feel they are acting in the best interest of the patient and not responding to their own internal curiosity or voyeuristic urges or, worse still, exploitation. If it is in response to a patient's request, for example, the search may be warranted. (However, looking at a patient's Facebook page or website may nonetheless most appropriately occur during a treatment session.) Clinton et al. (2010, p.104) cite the example of trying to locate the family of a hospitalized patient with dementia when all other efforts have failed. Safety concerns that most practitioners would agree constituted an emergency might provide another reasonable rationale for searching about a patient.

Unexpected findings can raise difficult ethical dilemmas that may warrant ethical consultation about whether to reveal the findings to the patient, report them to authorities, and/or document them in the medical record. In general, honesty and transparency seem important. Most relationships between health-care provider and patient can tolerate some breaches or disruptions if the fundamental alliance is in place. Knowing that a provider will be honest about such dilemmas may enhance rather than detract from the alliance.

Seeking the patient's explicit consent to search is often prudent, particularly if the provider feels that the patient's discovery of the search would compromise the treatment alliance. In such a case, the various options can be weighed together. For example, in the case of an adolescent who has reportedly expressed suicidal ideation or other unsafe behaviors on a Facebook page, looking at that page may be more tolerable to the adolescent than calling a parent or school personnel. Many times the search can be performed together, thus preserving the treatment frame.

Documenting the results of searches in the medical record is particularly complex in this era of electronic medical records (EMR) and unresolved dilemmas about who should have access to such records, use of cutting and pasting, and so on. Legal and ethical consultation may be warranted, and initial actions should err on the side of caution.

The need for continual monitoring of all of these questions is clear if the relationship is ongoing and the provider perceives a need for such searches. Particularly important to examine are the provider's feelings about the patient and the nature of the patient's feelings towards the provider. Ensuring that the frame remains in place and professional in nature is crucial.

11.5 SOCIAL MEDIA AND MEDIA-SHARING SITES

Unlike some other digital media, social media has official guidelines associated with its use in health care in the United States. Both the AMA and the FSMB issued guidelines about appropriate social media use. Here is a summary of the FSMB (2012) guidelines arranged in the six categories they offer:

1. **Interacting with patients** – Don't use personal social networking or social media sites such as Facebook to interact with patients. Any interactions should occur in the context of a physician–patient relationship. Be mindful that such interactions, while potentially helpful, can also detract from the quality of face-to-face interactions with the patient.

2. **Discussion of medicine online** – Professional interactions online can facilitate "peer-to-peer education and dialogue," (p. 7), but providers have responsibility, to the best of their ability, for ensuring security of such sites and that only verified and registered users can access the information. Websites should be password-protected, and any medical information that the provider intends to implement in practice needs to be varied from other sources of "current medical research" (p. 7). The guidelines cite the example of Doximity, a professional website with more than 567,000 physician members in 87 different specialties.

3. **Privacy/Confidentiality** – Patient privacy and confidentiality must be protected, per HIPAA. No information should be revealed that could potentially identify a patient, including room numbers, code names for patients, or pictures.

4. **Disclosure** – When writing online from the vantage point of a health-care professional, physicians are to reveal any potential conflicts of interest and be honest about their credentials.

5. **Posting content** – Here, providers are warned of the risks of postings being disseminated beyond the intended audience; remarks being taken out of context or misconstrued; and content being permanently accessible. They are asked to be professional. Employees of institutions are warned that employers may retain the right to "edit, modify, delete, or review Internet communications." They assume all security, privacy, and confidentiality risks of their own posts. Finally, if they are responsible for moderating websites, physicians are instructed to delete anything that is either inaccurate, violates patients' privacy and confidentiality or is of an unprofessional nature.

6. **Professionalism** – The FSMB offers the following general suggestions:

   - Use separate personal and professional social networking sites (e.g. use a personal email address for logging on to personal social media).
   - Report any observed unprofessional behavior to supervisory and/or regulatory authorities.
   - Adhere to the same professionalism principles online as offline.
   - Never engage in cyberbullying.
   - Refer to the employer's policy on social media and social networking for their use in the context of employment. (A case before the National Labor Relations Board decided that an employer could fire an employee for posting derogatory content about the practice as long as the employee was the only one posting such content; lots of employees posting content supposedly constitutes legitimate complaint [Dolan, 2011b]).

Finally, the FSMB guidelines warn that physicians may be subject to disciplinary action if their use of social media is unprofessional, including "inappropriate communication with patients online; use of the Internet for unprofessional behavior; online misrepresentation of credentials; online violations of patients confidentiality; failure to reveal conflicts of interests online; online derogatory remarks regarding a patient; online depiction of intoxication; discriminatory language or practices online" (FSMB, 2012, pp. 8–9). Disciplinary actions may range from a reprimand to having a license to practice revoked. As technology develops and social trends change ongoing behaviors and practice standards, the guidelines are expected to be updated.

The AMA (2010) guidelines are similar, although less developed. Regarding privacy they are perhaps more pragmatic: "Physicians should use privacy settings to safeguard personal information and content to the greatest extent possible, but should realize that privacy settings are not absolute and that once on the Internet, content is likely there permanently." Both FSMB and AMA guidelines may be incorporated in various ways into the regulations or guidelines of state medical boards across the country.

These guidelines, and others, recommend that health-care professionals should not respond to "friend" requests by patients. The blurring of personal and professional boundaries is simply too great. This boundary is an extension of the natural boundaries we already maintain – we don't invite our patients for drinks after a session, for example, or show them our most intimate possessions. In just the same way, we do not "friend" our patients on social media. However, managing the request can be delicate, and all efforts should be made to discuss that decision with the patient in a manner so as not to offend or shame. Ongoing monitoring of privacy settings is crucial, given the history of Facebook and others reverting to the default status (i.e. lowest privacy settings) without warning users ahead of time. For up-to-date information on how to set privacy settings on Facebook and Twitter, see their websites (Facebook, Help Centre-Privacy, www.facebook.com/help/?page-419; Twitter Help Centre, About public and protected accounts, support.twitter.com/entries/14016-about-public-and-protected-accounts).

Postings need to be cautious, and personal walls need to be surveyed regularly for content posted by others that may be compromising. A useful standard is the following: If a health-care provider wouldn't want a patient (or perhaps a respected relative) to see content, the best course is for the provider to delete it. Recall that any content can compromise one's defense in a malpractice suit since even private content can be accessed by litigation attorneys. Finally, if posting professional advice, avoid not only the appearance of a treatment relationship but also the appearance of a supervisory role (Vanderpool, 2012).

Our monitoring of inappropriate content does not only apply to ourselves: Both the FSMB guidelines and the AMA Policy on Professionalism in the Use of Social Media specifically states that if physicians find inappropriate content by other physicians online, they should bring that content to the attention of the other physician (see p. 144). If the latter does not take action to remove the inappropriate content, the AMA policy states that the matter should be reported to appropriate authorities (AMA, 2010).

Some medical practices have a professional Facebook page for the dissemination of information. For example, pediatrician Jennifer Thomas in Franklin, Wisconsin, is reported to run a small practice and manages two Facebook pages with a total of 4,000 followers (www.facebook.com/pages/Dr-Jen-4-Kids/195291585574). For such practices, experts advise preparing postings in advance and having a timed released. Some data suggests patients seek health information in the evening hours and consistent timing of postings is deemed helpful. Websites such as HootSuite and TweetDeck allow professionals to put together content ahead of time and then schedule when it will be automatically posted on Twitter. Other products allow postings within Facebook to be posted on Twitter, and vice versa (Dolan, 2011a). Undoubtedly, as technology develops, more similar tools will become available (see Chapter 12).

Other media-sharing sites, such as YouTube, are similar to Facebook with the difference that video opens the door even wider to potential patient-identifying information; hence the need for care is even more heightened. In this age of digitized visual content, virtually all videos and photographs can be transmitted to other sites.

CONCLUSION

Undoubtedly, digital technology and the Internet pose huge new opportunities for enhancing communication between health-care providers and related services and between providers and patients. However, to use these new technologies responsibly and professionally requires significant attention. Small practices that do not have the manpower to provide ongoing vigilance may refrain from much use of these technologies in their practices, although the trade-off may be a loss of patients/clients who are increasingly expecting and seeking such services in their health care. Larger practices may be able to hire personnel whose job it is to manage the technological aspects of the practice. All practitioners will inevitably need to include in their continuing medical education activities the acquisition of knowledge and skills around technology. These activities will require money, as will the technologies themselves. Paid consultation on an intermittent basis is likely also to be necessary. Because technology is likely to play an increasing role in how we practice, it can also be expected to take up an increasingly significant portion of our practice budgets.

But without becoming mired in technological details, health care professionals would do well to remember the fundamentals of professional online behavior:

- Use the most appropriate means of communication for a given task, including face-to-face.
- Learn how to use each means of communication safely and effectively.
- Know the policies and guidelines of your institution, licensing board, professional association, and malpractice insurer.
- Password-protect all devices.
- Set the frame ahead of time, preferably in writing, and adhere to it.
- Follow the rules of netiquette in all communications.
- Get consultation.
- Pay attention to issues of standard of care; patient confidentiality and security of patient information; patient and practitioner privacy; libel; disclosure of conflict of interest; academic integrity; and safety and mandated reporting requirements.

If these guidelines are followed, patients and practitioners may benefit from the many advantages of technology without compromising standards of professionalism.

REFERENCES

Adler, E.A. (2012). Text messaging and patients: Benefits and considerations. Retrieved from: <http://www.physicianspractice.com.text-messaging-and-patients-benefits-and-considerations>.

Alltucker, K. (2011). Scottsdale doctors awarded $12 million in defamation case. *Arizona Republic*, December 16. Retrieved from <http://bit.ly/17iwbxh>.

American Bar Association. (1999). Formal opinion No 99-413: Protecting the confidentiality of unencrypted e-mail. American Bar Association Standing Committee on Ethics and Professional Responsibility, March 10, 1999. Retrieved from <http://www.abanet.org>. Cited in Recupero (2005), p. 467.

American Medical Association. (1999). Guidelines for patient–physician electronic mail. Retrieved from <http://www.ama-assn.org/resources/doc/psa/x-ama/consultations.pdf>.

American Medical Association. (2010). Professionalism in the use of social media. Retrieved from <http://bit.ly/zpSrXf>.

American Psychological Association. (1997). APA statement on services by telephone, teleconferencing and Internet: A statement by the Ethics Committee of the American Psychological Association. Available from <www.apa.org>.

Atherton, H., Sawmynaden, P., Sheikh, A., Majeed, A., & Car, J. (2012). Email for clinical communication between patients/caregivers and healthcare professionals. Cochran Database of Systematic Reviews, Issue 11. Art No: CD007978. http://dx.doi.org/10.1002/14651858.CD007978.pub2.

Clinton, B. K., Silverman, B. C., & Brendel, D. H. (2010). Patient-targeted googling: The ethics of searching online for patient information. *Harvard Review of Psychiatry, 18*, 103–112.

Dolan, P.L. (2011a). A few simple tricks can improve social media postings. Technically speaking. *American Medical News*, May 23. Retrieved from <http://www.ama-assn.org/amednews/2011/05/23/bica0523.htm>.

Dolan, P.L. (2011b). NLRB report raises questions about social media use at practices. *American Medical News*, September 26. Retrieved from <www.ama-assn.org/amednews/2011/09/26/bica0926.htm>.

Dolan, P.L. (2012). How to ensure a lost mobile device won't cause a data breach. *American Medical News/Business*, March 26. Retrieved from <http://www.ama-assn.org/amednews/2012/03/26/bica0326.htm>.

Eysenbach, G. (2000). Towards ethical guidelines for dealing with unsolicited patient emails and giving teleadvice in the absence of a pre-existing patient–physician relationship – Systematic review and expert survey. *Journal of Medical Internet Research, 2*(1), e1. Retrieved from <http://www.jmir.org/2000/1/e1/>.

Farrell, M.B. (2012). A low profile – Boston start-up joins those that will try to help you keep personal data off the Web. *The Boston Globe*, Business/Science and Innovation, July 23.

Federation of State Medical Boards, Inc. (FSMB) (2002). Model guidelines for the appropriate use of the Internet in medical practice. Retrieved from <http://www.fsmb.org/pdf/2002_grpol_use_of_internet.pdf>.

Federation of State Medical Boards, Inc. (FSMB) (2012). Model policy guidelines for the appropriate use of social media and social networking in medical practice. Retrieved from <www.fsmb.org/pdf/pub-social-media-guidelines.pdf>.

Fogg, B. D., & Eckles, D. (Eds). (2007). *Mobile persuasion: 20 perspectives of the future of behavior change*. Palo Alto, CA: Stanford Captology Media.

Hoffman, J.K. (2012). Texting the teenage patient, *The New York Times*, Oct 8.

Huntley, A. C. (1999). The need to know: Patients, e-mail and the Internet. *Archives of Dermatology, 135*(2), 198–199. http://dx.doi.org/10.1001/archderm.135.2.198.

Jones S. (2009). Generations online in 2009. Pew Research Center's Internet & American Life Project. Retrieved from <http://www.pewinternet.org/Reports/2009/Generations-Online-in-2009.aspx>.

Kane, B., & Sands, D. Z. (1998). Guidelines for the clinical use of electronic mail with patients. *Journal of the American Medical Informatics Association, 5*, 104–111. http://dx.doi.org/10.1136/jamia.1998.0050104.

Lee, T.B. (2011). Patient sues dentist over gag order; gets Medical Justice to backtrack. Law and Disorder/Civilization and discontents. Retrieved from <arstechnica.com>, <http://ars.to/Mp8bAF>.

Lewis, A. D. (2000). Patients, physicians, and e-mail [letter reply]. *Archives of Dermatology, 136*(1), 121–122.

Maheu, M., & Gordon, B. (2000). Counseling and therapy on the Internet. *Professional Psychology: Research and Practice, 31*(5), 484–489.

Mostaghimi, A., Crotty, B. H., & Landono, B. E. (2010). The availability and nature of physician information on the internet. *Journal of General Internal Medicine, 25*, 1152–1156.

Recupero, P. (2005). Email and the psychiatrist–patient relationship. *Journal of the American Academy of Psychiatry and the Law, 33*, 465–467.

Reents S., & Miller, T.E. (1998). The health care industry in transition – The online mandate to change. Cyber Dialogue. Retrieved from <http://www.cyberdialogue.com/free_data/white_papers/intel_health_day.html>.

Richmond, R. (2011). How to fix (or kill) web data about you. *The New York Times*, April 13, 2011. Retrieved from <http://nyti.ms/17LTMI1>.

Segal, J., (2012) Managing your online reputation. Greenbranch Publishing LLC. Retrieved from <www.greenbranch.com>.

Sims, H., Sanghara, H., Hayes, D., Wandiembe, S., Finch, M., Jakobsen, H., et al. (2012). Text message reminders of appointments: A pilot intervention at four community mental health clinics in London. *Psychiatric Services, 63,* 161–168.

Singer, N. (2012). Your digital Switzerland – An entrepreneur builds a virtual vault to secure personal data. *The New York Times*, December.

Tehrani, A., Feldman, S., Camacho, F., & Balkirshnan, R. (2011). Patient satisfaction with outpatient medical care in the United States. *Health Outcomes Research in Medicine, 2,* e197–e202.

Terry, M. (2008). Text messaging in healthcare: The elephant knocking at the door. *Telemedicine and e-Health*, July-August 2008, http://dx.doi.org/10.1089/tmj.2008.8495.

Vanderpool, D. (2012, May). Technology in psychiatry: Managing the risks. New England Council of Child and Adolescent Psychiatry, Early Career Psychiatrist Conference, Waltham, MA.

Welfel, E.R., & Bunce, R. (2003). How psychologists use e-mail with current clients: A national survey. Poster presented at the annual meeting of the American Psychological Association. Cited in Drude, K., Lichstein, M. (2002), *Psychologists use of e-mail with clients: Some ethical considerations*. Retrieved from <kspope.com/ethics/email.php>.

Zickuhr, K. (2012). Digital differences. Pew Research Center's Internet & American Life Project. Retrieved from <http://www.pewinternet.org/Presentations/2012/Oct/WSU-Digital-Differences.aspx>.

Chapter | Twelve

The Future of Technology in Health Care

"Luddites" were nineteenth-century British anti-industrialists who destroyed factories and machines to protest against the sweeping changes of the Industrial Revolution. However, voicing caution about using technology in health care does not make one a Luddite. The Digital Revolution may elicit such tendencies in some who fear change or a loss of humanism in medicine, or in those whom it makes feel incompetent and obsolete. The inclination to respond to technological innovations with a "Just say no" approach may be tempting. Perhaps particularly in this dichotomous age where black-and-white thinking often seems to prevail (technology is "all good" or "all bad"), defining a middle-ground position can be difficult. But in fact, a middle-ground position is what health care needs to assume.

Technology is here to stay and offers health care enormous opportunities to improve care for patients. It also poses significant professionalism risks, especially when technology is at the interface between provider and patient. The overarching dilemma for health-care practitioners is how to integrate technological innovations into health-care practice without jeopardizing the professionalism standards discussed in this book. In this chapter, the potential for technology in health-care will be examined with an emphasis on the real public good that can come from its use.

In his influential book, cardiologist and technology advocate Eric Topol (2012) argues that what is needed is the "creative destruction of medicine." Thanks to what he calls a superconvergence of innovations like wireless sensors, genomics, imaging techniques, data-gathering and computational systems, mobile connectivity and increased bandwidth,

S. deJong: Blogs and Tweets, Texting and Friending.
DOI: http://dx.doi.org/10.1016/B978-0-12-408128-4.00012-6
© 2014 S. DeJong. Published by Elsevier Inc. All rights reserved.

and social networking and the Internet, a "new medicine" that puts technology at the forefront for both patients and providers lies within our grasp (p. vii). However, Topol argues, conservatism in the medical profession and, he implies, the medical establishment's concerns about losing power and income due to technology, mean that change will need to be pushed through by consumers. This argument is essentially an extension of the "power-to-the-people" approach of crowd-sourcing, which started with the realization that highly skilled jobs performed by an employee could be outsourced to an online workforce. Thus entities such as Wikipedia (the online, publicly authored encyclopedia) and Threadless.com for T-shirt design provide methods for inexpensive innovation that places power at the hands of the online user. Today, major scientific contests are held online, such as General Electric's breast cancer challenge. Most recently, with the advent of online genetic data, even gene therapies and viral methods for delivering them are now crowd-sourced. Those like Topol who are advocating for technology in medicine are also arguing for power to the patient; that is, using technology to put patients more in charge of their own health care, including advocating for professionals to adopt helpful technologies.

Undoubtedly, the rate of growth in information technology is exponential and, as costs continue to decrease, integrating technology into clinical practice is becoming a reality. With extraordinary prescience, Intel co-founder Gordon Moore noted in 1965 that computer chips were doubling in capacity (number of integrated circuits) every year and predicted they would go on to do so for a decade. In fact, his prediction has held for 50 years, is now known as "Moore's Law," and applies broadly to the rate of all technological development: Internet data, computer storage bytes per dollar, digital-camera pixels per dollar, data transfer capacity of optical fibers, and so on, all appear to double each year. Thus, the most powerful computers of the 1970s, which took up whole rooms and cost millions of dollars to manufacture, have given way to the smartphones of today which are "100 times faster and more than 12,000 times cheaper … This is exponential growth at work" (Hessel, Goodman & Kotler, 2012, p. 4).

Many of these technologies offer opportunities for improving health care without jeopardizing professionalism. The availability and rapid transfer of general health-care information online mean that better-informed patients can participate more actively in their care. Manhattan Research reports that 79% of patients with chronic diseases use the Internet to help them make decisions about their care, up from 53% in 2011 (Dolan, P.L., 2012). Online reminders about appointments (provided by services like DoctorConnect.net and patientnudge.com in the USA) and medications can improve patient compliance (Spielmans, 2012). Online reminders to physicians about required clinical practices such as end-of-care planning have the potential to improve care (Abrams, 2013). Sensors collecting a vast array of biodata (the iHealth movement) mean that health-care professionals can have more complete and representative data on which to base medical decision-making.

Many of these technologies are already being used in practice to monitor clinical problems. Examples of such problems include pain management in cancer patients (Dempster, Bewick Jones & Bennett, 2012); cognitive rehabilitation in patients with chronic neurologic conditions (Seelye, Schmitter-Edgecombe, Das & Cook, 2012); coordination of home-based care (Morishima & Kijima, 2012); and lifestyle and behavioral modifications in patients with obesity (Bacigalupo et al., 2012). The remote management of chronic medical conditions is the function of the majority of mobile apps that have been approved to date by the Food and Drug Administration in the US, with EKG-monitoring the next most common (Dolan, B., 2012).

But as psychiatrist Joel Yager points out in his paper on the future of technology in psychiatry, paradigm shifts occur at a rate determined by factors other than (or perhaps in addition to) professional inertia and self-interest: "Scientific advances are implemented only at the pace that social–cultural shifts and economic realities permit. Today's marvelous discoveries may take decades to work into common practice, depending on providers and practitioner acceptance, utility, and financing" (Yager, 2011). Yager points to the slow and scattered adoption of the electronic medical record as an example.

However, there can be little doubt that the democratization of health care via technology is underway and may well lead to the increase in consumer demand for health-care providers to embrace technology that Topol envisions. Online patient networks such as PatientsLikeMe provide a forum for patients who share a diagnoses to compare notes and get support (Topol, 2012, p. x). Crowd-sourcing techniques are being used to develop new health-care technologies. Consider the example, cited in Adler (2012, p. 3), of Health Tech Hatch, which "invites online users to use their smartphones to develop videos that can be used in health care":

> *Pathfinders Medical is partnering with Health Tech Hatch, a new health-focused crowdfunding site that supports the growth of new technologies that will make healthcare better for all of us... We would like to extend an invitation to "join the crowd" to help make this video library a reality.*

At least six categories of technological innovation are poised for revolutionizing health care in productive ways: sensors, imaging devices, genetics, supercomputing and "big data" synthesis, robotics, and energy harvesting. Let us look at how these are already starting to change health care.

Thanks in part to the fitness movement, wireless sensors that measure individuals' vital signs, blood sugar, and other physiological parameters have become so commonplace, the notion of "the quantified self" has entered popular parlance. This data can be collected and communicated to health-care professionals via mobile phones. Global sales of such "mobile-health apps" were estimated to grow from $718 million in 2011 to $1.3 billion in 2012 (*The Economist*, 2012b, p. 13).

In the spirit of Star Trek's tricorder, which allowed Dr. McCoy to diagnose the damage inflicted on Captain Kirk by an alien, health-care professionals and inventors aspire to have sensors that can be used for diagnosis (*The Economist*, 2012b, p. 12). In 2012, Qualcomm, a manufacturer of wireless communication devices, announced the "Tricorder XPrize" of $10 million that has received applications from 230 teams in 30 different countries. The "tricorder" must be a mobile platform that permits the diagnosis of 15 different conditions (e.g. diabetes, sleep apnea) without the presence of a doctor or a nurse. Companies such as Nokia and Qualcomm are putting venture capital into start-ups like San Francisco's AliveCor, which has developed an electrode-containing iPhone case that can perform an electrocardiogram.

Increasingly mobile devices are being used as medical and laboratory instruments. AgaMatrix has developed a way to provide long-term glucose monitoring for patients with diabetes using test strips and an iPhone (*The Economist*, 2012b, p. 13). The CellScope turns the phone into a microscope that can be used to examine the retina for the presence of pathogens such as malaria and tuberculosis and an otoscope for detecting ear infections (p. 14). The Zeo clock functions as an electroencephalograph, sensing brainwaves during sleep (Topol, 2012, pp. 63–64). In the near future, nanosensors implanted in the body may be programed to scan for cancer cells and myocardial infarction (Topol, 2012, pp. 162–165).

Imaging of organs is another area of technological opportunity. Organs such as the heart can be imaged using sound waves. An ultrasonic probe developed by MobiSante, and FDA-approved in 2011, can be plugged into a mobile phone to create an image (*The Economist* 2012b, p. 14). Topol described using the Vscan to image his own heart, and voiced the opinion that the instrument was going to replace the stethoscope (Topol, pp. 122–123). Technology is also used, of course, to image the brain through MRIs and fMRIs and to provide neurologic treatments through everything from electroconvulsive therapy to deep brain stimulation. Moreover, imaging is also used to measure the effect of drugs such as anticancer agents. The advent of 3-D imaging promises to open up more opportunities, and "organ printing" is on its way.

Third in the list of major technological innovations is rapid genetic sequencing, an area of skyrocketing growth thanks to decreasing costs of the technology. While the first genome sequence took 13 years and $2.7 billion, the 2007 genome project led by Craig Venter took 4 years and around $100 million, and, currently, companies like Complete Genomics can sequence about a thousand human genomes a month for a few thousand dollars each (Topol, p. 95). Hospitals such as Massachusetts General now offer "whole genome sequencing and interpretation service for patients" (Tornsho, 2013, p. 8). "Chip medicine," (You on a chip), has become a reality and celebrities from Glenn Close to Stephen Pinker have publicized their genomic findings.

Can genomic sequencing result in successful therapies? In 2010 the case of Nicholas Volker, a 5-year-old with a rare gastrointestinal disorder that proved to be the result of a mutation in the gene XIAP, was the first case of reported genetic treatment and resulted in health insurances agreeing to cover genetic therapies. Genome-wide association studies have opened the door to how medications interact with specific genes. They have aided in unveiling drugs' therapeutic actions and in predicting treatment responses to medications such as the blood thinner warfarin (Topol, pp. 89–91). Similar studies looking at correlates between gene variants and the risk of heart disease, cancer, diabetes, asthma, and other illnesses are helping us understand why, to whom, and when such diseases happen (Topol, 2012, pp. 160–170). The application of supercomputer technology to human genome sequencing is expected to decrease processing times exponentially to mere minutes and make the digital sequencing of most human conditions soon within reach (Rothberg, 2011). Authors like Topol argue that genetic access should be democratized and that "routine molecular biologic digitization of humankind is just around the corner" (Topol, 2012, p. 121).

Genetics is just one example of a pool of information to which new "big data" mining and synthesis can be applied. Just as businesses have used data mining to track consumer behaviors, health-care professionals have used it to learn about health patterns (Talbot, 2011). By surveying online users' Tweets and Google searches, headache researchers have acquired data about timing of migraine episodes (Linman, Maleki, Becerra & Borsook, 2013). Similar research on mental health queries made on Google between 2006 and 2010 in the US and Australia found seasonal differences in the rates of specific mental health diagnoses (Ayers, Althouse, Allern Rosenquist & Ford, 2013). Applying big data analyses to electronic medical records offers the potential to more sensitively detect medication side-effects and complications from medical devices than the current voluntary reporting system currently employed by the Food and Drug Administration in the US. For example, in the nationalized health-care system of Sweden, scanning data in the national database provided insight into liver toxicity occurring at a rate of 1% in patients treated with a new anticoagulant (Lagerqvist, 2004).

Computers with a capacity for big-data synthesis can be placed in robots located in the clinical setting. For example, the Sloane-Kettering Hospital in New York is training the famous IBM Watson supercomputer (the one that defeated two human champions on Jeopardy) to digest and synthesize medical information at a rate of up to 60 million pages of text per second with the goal of improving diagnostic accuracy.

Another application of robots in medicine are "telepresence robots." These remotely controlled, mobile devices offer a less expensive version of video-conferencing. The wheeled robot is equipped with a camera, microphone, loudspeaker, and screen that displays the face of the remote operator. Such a robot, "driven" by a supervisor, might accompany an intern on ward rounds to provide advice and consultation. Companies such as RoboDynamics of Santa Monica, CA, have reportedly sold more than 100 of its TILR robots since 2008 for a price of $10,000 each. The technology is so effective, the Brazilian Olympic Organizing Committee is planning on putting robots in operating rooms for the 2016 games so that athletes' medical care can be supervised by their regular physicians at home (*The Economist*, 2012a, p. 11).

Finally, robots are being used in surgical procedures. Dr. Douglas Murphy, a cardiac surgeon at St. Joseph's Hospital in Atlanta, used a robot in repairing mitral valves and his hospital has launched the International College of Robotic Surgery (Salter, 2009, p. 4). The Da Vinci robotic surgery system, FDA approved for soft-tissue surgery, was used to perform more than 40,000 (half the annual total) of prostate removals in 2008 (Salter, p. 6).

The sixth and last major technological innovation likely to have significant applicability to health care is energy harvesting. The concept behind energy harvesting is that the energy generated from the body's natural processes (e.g. a beating heart, skeletal muscle flexion, and contraction) can be "harvested" and then used to wirelessly provide enough energy to drive implanted devices such as cardiac pacemakers. Because the energy can be stored, the pacemaker can keep the heart beating even after a myocardial infarction until an external defibrillator can be used (*The Economist*, 2012c).

These six developing technologies, together with those already existing, such as electronic medical records, email, social media, and so on, are likely to transform medical encounters of the future.

Technological obstacles such as protecting privacy and device security are likely to be addressed by newer technological innovations. An example of technology healing itself is "Snapchat" which allows users to send messages and photos that then disappear in a few seconds. As Snapchat founder Evan Spiegel is quoted as saying, "It became clear how awful social media is. There is real value in sharing moments that don't live forever" (Wortham, 2013). Technology is a rapidly advancing frontier, with problems being identified and solved in rapid succession. Improved encryption techniques, secure text messages that automatically download into the medical record – these are examples of technological solutions to technological problems that are on their way.

Already, large health organizations such as The Mayo Clinic in Minnesota and Kaiser Permanente in California are embracing technology system-wide. Mayo, for example, opened a new Center for Social Media with more than 60,000 followers on Twitter and 20,000 Facebook connections. Lee Aase, the CEO of Mayo, reported to the *Wall Street Journal* that the Center's goal was "To help patients. Sometimes that means providing information directly to them, and sometimes it means disseminating information more rapidly to the medical community" (Health Blog Q&A, 2010, cited in Topol, 2012, p. 190).

What will health care look like in the future? Writing for Fast Company in 2009, journalist Chuck Salter describes the "The Doctor of the Future," Dr. Jay Parkinson. Parkinson, a recent graduate of Johns Hopkins' pediatric training program, started a virtual practice in Brooklyn in 2007 using a website, blog, house calls, and e-visits. Though he did not accept insurance (payment was through PayPal), three hundred patients joined his practice in the first three months. When the media publicized his practice, he was "discovered" by Canadian entrepreneur Nathaniel Findlay, CEO of software company Myca Health, which had developed a platform for mobile telemedicine. Findlay invited Parkinson to become his chief concept officer. The Myca platform's functions include electronic medical records, a practice-management component, and a social-networking site with doctor and patient photos and profiles, all with enough security to meet federal privacy standards.

Patients who use Myca choose a medical team based on providers' profiles, make appointments (face-to-face, video, or instant messaging) on the doctor's schedule, and fill out a textbox describing their chief complaint. For physicians, the platform provides access to the appointment calendar, medication refill requests, a "snapshot" of conditions treated in the local area that week, and the capacity to email all patients with a given disorder to provide new information and reminders (Salter, 2009, pp. 3–4).

The future will also bring the capacity for quick consultation with professional peers. Software systems such as SimulConsult, Isabel, and Diagnosaurus provide rapid problem-solving about diagnostic and other clinical problems for physicians in real time. The clinical reach is likely to become global as health-care professionals provide supervision to underserved areas around the world, limited only by trade barriers and licensing restrictions. Patients will likewise be comparing notes and seeking answers from each other through sites such as PatientsLikeMe (Salter, 2009).

These changes are all likely to significantly alter health-care education. Already, traditional lecture-hall teaching has been supplanted by online learning modalities. Even clinical learning can occur at a distance thanks to "virtualized" laboratories and telesupervision (Yager, 2011, p. 284). Student–faculty interactions (just like those between provider and patients) are likely to become increasingly asynchronous: Health-care education can take place anywhere, anytime. Students themselves are using social media platforms to engage in peer-to-peer teaching and consultation, like the ScholarLocker site developed by Harvard medical students. Health-care students of the future can expect to be evaluated on their skills using the new technologies, including their ability to connect with patients "virtually" (Srinivasan, Keenan & Yager, 2006).

While all these extraordinary innovations do mean that health care is poised for radical change, intellectual historian Thomas Kuhn (author of the classic book *The Structure of Scientific Revolutions*) reminds us that scientific and technological paradigms do not move neatly from one to the next. He notes that while paradigm shifts occur in the context of a crisis (which current health-care costs certainly constitute), scientists may "begin to lose faith and consider alternatives," but they "do not renounce the paradigm that has led them into crisis" until they find a suitable replacement (Kuhn, 1970, p. 77).

What are the obstacles to moving from current health-care practices to the efficient, accessible, and hopefully cost-effective technologically driven health-care system that Topol and others envision? The history of the digital revolution demonstrates that technological changes are innovated and embraced initially by pioneers, often youthful ones. (Interestingly, Kuhn (1970, p. 90) notes that "almost always, the men who achieve … fundamental inventions of a new paradigm have been very young or very new to the field whose paradigm they change.") Thus the Mark Zuckerbergs and Jay Parkinsons lead the way and others follow at varying speeds, depending on interest level, cultural values, economic incentives, access, and other factors. In the case of health care, as many have noted, the culture has tended to be one of caution. Caution towards the wholesale adoption of technological innovation appears in part well-founded.

Health-care professionals may be cautious, and even skeptical, about technological innovations, in part because of what the IT firm Gartner termed "the hype cycle:" A new technology is introduced with much fanfare and enthusiasm. When its promise is not immediately realized, a "trough of disillusionment" sets in. This trough may last varying amounts of time before being followed by the upward "slope of enlightenment" as inevitable kinks are worked out. Thus, over time, many innovations do take hold but in the short-term may be slowed down as unforeseen problems are resolved. One example might be the advent of electronic medical records. While heralded with the promise of increased efficiency, fewer medical errors, and lower costs, such results have not been consistently demonstrated, and many health care professionals might argue that they have a long way to go before becoming user-friendly. However, systems such as the Veterans Health Administration and the health-care firm Kaiser Permanente are devoted to making electronic records work and are already coming up with more successful models (Topol, 2012, pp. 148–150).

Another deterrent to embracing technology is the concern that regulation consistently lags behind innovation. Particularly in the US, technology has developed largely in the free market, unfettered by government restriction. While free-market supporters may argue that such an environment fosters healthy innovation, the lack of oversight concerns others. For example, writing in *The Atlantic*, authors Hessel, Goodman & Kotler (2012) imagine a world of bio-design websites in which consumers can upload their disease information and a virologist could develop a customized cure: "What people did with these bio-designs was anybody's guess. No international body had yet been created to watch over them" (p. 1). They cite *The New York Times* commentary on the International Genetically Engineered Machine (iGEM) competition started by MIT in 2004:

> *iGEM has been grooming an entire generation of the world's brightest scientific minds to embrace synthetic biology's vision – without anyone really noticing, before the public debates and regulations that typically place checks on such risky and ethically controversial new technologies have even started"* (pp. 8–9).

A major thrust of these authors' concern is that while new technological innovations may be directed towards prosocial ends, they may equally be employed by terrorists and criminals for antisocial activities. Antisocial behaviors range from the activities of "Mafiaboy," a Canadian high-school student who all by himself succeeded in slowing down or freezing Amazon, Dell, CNN, eBay, and Yahoo websites (Hessel, Goodman & Kotler, 2012, p. 9) to the activities of organized crime. (In Japan, the *yakuza* now outsources its murders to hitmen in Chinese gangs.) Nations such as China appear to be using the Internet to exert control rather than promote freedom (*The Economist*, 2013). While no one is likely to argue that health-care professionals who embrace technology are going to turn into terrorists, such stories may reinforce their hesitation to do so.

Like all innovations in health care, evidence is needed to determine whether new technological devices and software systems are in fact helpful to patients. The need for evidence is particularly important given the initial hype, described above, when a new product is released, as well as the concerning lack of critical thinking skills suggested by those studying plagiarism in academic environments (see Chapter 9). As noted earlier, the evidence regarding electronic medical records has been disappointing: For example, a 2009 study from the University of Minnesota examined four years of Medicare data to discover whether IT applications such as EMRs, nurse charts, and picture arching and communications systems (PACS) had improved three patient safety indicators: infection due to medical care; postoperative hemorrhage or hematoma; and postoperative pulmonary embolism or deep vein thrombosis. The authors reported finding "little evidence that IT improved quality" (Parente & McCullough, 2009, p. 358).

In most areas of medicine, the evidence for and against new technologies is mixed: Efforts to use email to encourage lifestyle changes have run into difficulties in getting patients to initiate and maintain their use of online tools (Gold, 2013). A study of smartphone applications for monitoring suspicious skin moles found mixed reliability (Wolf, Moreau, Akilov, et al., 2013). In addition, a 2013 study in the *British Medical Journal* of remote vital-sign monitoring for 1,500 patients with chronic illness failed to find any significant health, quality of life or psychological benefits (Cartwright, Hirani, Rixon, et al., 2013); moreover, the cost of care by tele-health was higher than that for usual care (Henderson, Knapp, Fernandez, et al., 2013).

On the other side of the evidence balance are studies supporting the efficacy of technological interventions. For example, one study found that epilepsy patients show improved treatment adherence when they can connect to other patients through PatientsLikeMe (Hall, 2013). A number of studies indicate the effectiveness of online interventions for the detection and management of mental health disorders in primary care (Reid, Kauser, Hearps, et al., 2011; Roy-Byrne, Craske, Sullivan, et al., 2010). The mixed nature of the evidence overall underscores the need for ongoing rigorous assessment of whether technology truly improves patient care.

As suggested by the BMJ study cited above, cost is a significant issue in the incorporation of technology into health care. While large health-care systems such as Kaiser Permanente and the US Veterans Administration may take advantage of economies of scale to make technological implementations cost-effective, smaller systems and, certainly, individual practitioners may find that technology's cost outweighs its benefits. Health care providers of the future may find that considerable time and money is needed in order to harness the advantages of technology. Examples such as Dr. Jay Parkinson and the Myca Platform discussed above raise related concerns about access: If the technological pioneers do not take insurance, as Dr. Parkinson did not, technological advances may be further restricted to boutique practices rather than mainstream care.

The digital revolution has disrupted the conventional practice of medicine already and will continue to do so through the advances discussed above. In our free-market system, advances are likely to continue relatively unfettered, with regulatory bodies and ethical overseers racing to keep up. Hype about new technologies risks overshadowing evidence-based truths about their clinical efficacy. But thanks to technology itself, many kinks in new devices and software programs are likely to be solved over time, and we will ultimately move to a health-care system in which technology plays a prominent role in diagnosis, treatment, research, and education.

Today we live in a messy transitional zone between two paradigms. Some practitioners and systems are out ahead of the crowd, rapidly adopting technological innovations. Many lag behind. Still others will choose never to join the digital revolution. If we are confused by the state of affairs, imagine what it must feel like from the patients' perspective. While we navigate this transition, it is especially important that health-care providers adhere to the principles of professionalism outlined in this book while remaining curious about the real opportunities that technology will inevitably bring to our patients, and be willing to incorporate new technologies into practice when evidence suggests that doing so is feasible and likely to benefit those for whom we care. Ultimately, technology will play a critical role in the professional practice of medicine.

REFERENCES

Abrams, L. (2013). When doctors need e-mail reminders to talk to patients about death. *The Atlantic*. Downloaded from <http://bit.ly/103596W>.

Adler, L. (2012). Help us help you turn your smartphone into a healthcare advocate. Hatchlink. Retrieved from <http://www.thedoctorweighsin.com/?s= help-us-help-you-turn-your+smartphone>.

Ayers, J. W., Althouse, B. M., Allern, J. -P., Rosenquist, J. N., & Ford, D. E. (2013). Seasonality in seeking mental health information on Google. *American Journal of Preventive Medicine, 44*(5), 520–525.

Bacigalupo, R., Cudd, P., Littlewood, C., Bissell, P., Hawley, M. S., & Buckley Woods, H. (2012). Interventions employing mobile technology for overweight and obesity: An early systematic review of randomized controlled trials. *Obesity Reviews*. http://dx.doi.org/10.1111/obr.12006.

Cartwright, M., Hirani, S. P., Rixon, L., Beynon, M., Doll, H., Bower, P., et al. (2013). Effect of telehealth on quality of life and psychological outcomes over 12 months (Whole Systems Demonstrator telehealth questionnaire study): Nested study of patient reported outcomes in a pragmatic, cluster randomized controlled trial. *British Medical Journal, 346*, f653. http://dx.doi.org/10.1136/bmj/f653

Dempster, P. G., Bewick, B. M., Jones, R., & Bennett, M. I. (2012). Management of cancer pain in the community: Perceptions of current UK information technology systems and implications for future development. *Health Informatics, 18*(4), 284–293.

Dolan, B. (2012). Analysis: 75 FDA-cleared mobile medical apps. *Mobihealthnews*, December 20. Retrieved from <http://bit.ly/12C7GJg>.

Dolan, P.L. (2012). Patients online drill deep for information on doctors, procedures. *American Medical News*, November 5. Retrieved from <http://bit.ly/10VBVyl>.

Gold, A. (2013). E-mail prompts spur activity in online lifestyle intervention programs. FierceHealthIT. Retrieved from <www.fiercehealthitcom/node/18928/print>.

Hall, S.D. (2013). Social networks improve research, help patients with regimen adherence. FierceHealthIT February 12. Retrieved from <www.fiercehealthitcom/node/18983>.

HealthBlog Q&A, (2010). Mayo Clinic's new center for social media. *Wall Street Journal*, July 27. Retrieved from <http://on.wsj.com/aBwwUg>. Cited in Topol (2012).

Henderson, C., Knapp, M., Fernandez, J. -L., et al. (2013). Cost effectiveness of telehealth for patients with long term conditions (Whole Systems Demonstrator telehealth questionnaire study): Nested economic evaluation in a pragmatic, cluster randomized controlled trial. *British Medical Journal*, *346*, f1035. http://dx.doi.org/10.1136/bmj.f1035.

Hessel, A., Goodman, M., & Kotler S. (2012). Hacking the president's DNA. *The Atlantic*. Retrieved from <http://bit.ly/PRKEeT>.

Kuhn, T. (1970). *The structure of scientific revolutions* (2nd ed.). Chicago, IL: University of Chicago Press.

Lagerqvist, B. (2004). Is that it, then, for blockbuster drugs? *Lancet*, *365* 9440, 1100.

Linnman, C., Maleki, N., Becerra, L., & Borsook, D. (2013). Migraine tweets – What can online behavior tell us about disease? *Cephalalgia*, *33*(1), 68–69.

Morishima, A., & Kijima, Y. (2012). Sharing patient information using iPads in the introduction of IT for home medical care – Construction of a network for home care. *Gan To Kagaku Ryoho*, *39*(12), 6–8.

Parente, S. T., & McCullough, J. S. (2009). Health information technology and patient safety: Evidence from panel data. *Health Affairs*, *28*, 357–360.

Reid, S. C., Kauser, S. D., Hearps, S. J. C., Crooke, A. H. D., Khor, A. S., Sanci, L. A., et al. (2011). A mobile phone application for the assessment and management of youth mental health problems in primary care – a RTTC. *BMC Family Practice*, *12*, 131. Retrieved from <wwwmedscape.com/viewarticle/757714_print>.

Rothberg, J. M. (2011). An integrated semiconductor device enabling nonoptical genome sequencing. *Nature*, *475*, 348–352.

Roy-Byrne, P., Craske, M. G., Sullivan, G., et al. (2010). Delivery of evidence-based treatment for multiple anxiety disorders in primary care: A randomized, controlled trial. *Journal of the American Medical Association*, *303*, 1921–1928.

Salter, C. (2009). *Leadership: The doctor of the future*. Retrieved from <http://www.fastcompany.com/1266043/doctor-future>.

Seelye, A. M., Schmitter-Edgecombe, M., Das, B., & Cook, D. J. (2012). Application of cognitive rehabilitation theory to the development of smart prompting technologies. *IEEE Reviews in Biomedical Engineering*, *5*, 29–44.

Spielmans, G. (2012). Research updates in psychiatry. *The Carlat Psychiatry Report*, *10*(6), 6.

Srinivasan, M., Keenan, C. R., & Yager, J. (2006). Visualizing the future: Technology competency development in clinical medicine, and implications for medical education. *Academic Psychiatry*, *30*(6), 480–490.

Talbot, D. (2011). A social-media decoder. *Technology Review*, November–December, 44–51.

The Economist, (2012a). Your alter ego on wheels. *The Economist*, December 15–17, Technology Quarterly, pp. 11–12.

The Economist, (2012b). The dream of the medical tricorder. *The Economist*, December 15–17, Technology Quarterly, pp. 12–14.

The Economist, (2012c). Let's have a heart to heart. *The Economist*, December 15–17, Technology Quarterly, p. 6, 7.

The Economist, (2013). Special report: China and the Internet – A giant cage. *The Economist*, April 6–12, pp. 1–15.

Topol, E. (2012). *The creative destruction of medicine*. New York, NY: Basic Books.

Tornsho, R. (2013). Big data's powerful promise. *MassGeneral Magazine*, Winter 2013, pp. 8–13.

Wolf, J. A., Moreau, J. F., Akilov, O., et al. (2013). Diagnostic inaccuracy of smartphone applications for melanoma detection. *JAMA Dermatology*, *149*(4), 422–426. http://dx.doi.org/10.1001/jamadermatol.2013.2382.

Wortham, J. (2013). A growing app lets you see it, then you don't. *The New York Times*, February 8. Retrieved from: <http://nyti.ms/129NqfO>.

Yager, J. (2011). The practice of psychiatry in the 21st century: Challenges for psychiatric education. *Academic Psychiatry*, *35*(5), 285.

Chapter | Thirteen

Conclusion

Professionalism embodies qualities of the health-care clinician, that clinician's care of individual patients, and the clinician's relationships to students, peers, and society as a whole. It includes individual attributes such as altruism and self-reflection; clinical attributes such as expertise and adherence to ethical standards; and professional relationships characterized by respect, trust, and social responsibility.

Boundaries are an integral part of professionalism. Implicit boundaries circumscribe our relationships with patients, hospitals, and academic institutions, and our profession. They represent a limit of acceptable behavior. Boundaries also describe a protection from outside intrusion (as in confidential information and personal privacy), and the need to separate certain roles or else disclose potential conflicts. Many professionalism breaches involve some transgression of boundaries.

Social media and the Internet provide new avenues for breaches of professionalism. Digital technologies have distinctive features that make such breaches particularly concerning: They are easily accessible, mobile, and used globally across socioeconomic, demographic, and professional groups. They disseminate information with unprecedented speed and scope. Their content, unless protected by encryption or other devices, lacks confidentiality and security but is largely permanent. Our use of technology is not compartmentalized by place, time or audience (personal or professional). Textual content lacks nonverbal cues and is subject to misinterpretation. Finally, digital technologies change so rapidly, digital immigrants are constantly racing to keep up, and the rate of change out-paces the capacity of regulatory bodies to set appropriate standards. As Marshall McLuhan reminds us, media themselves, not just their message, have social consequences. Digital media have not only transformed society but also altered

S. deJong: Blogs and Tweets, Texting and Friending.
DOI: http://dx.doi.org/10.1016/B978-0-12-408128-4.00013-8
© 2014 S. DeJong. Published by Elsevier Inc. All rights reserved.

fundamental concepts of professionalism, including privacy and intellectual property.

This book has focused on eight broad categories in which professionalism issues can arise in the use of digital technology: liability and maintaining the standard of care; confidentiality and security of patient information; patient and practitioner privacy; libel; conflict of interest; academic honesty, particularly plagiarism; mandated reporting and safety issues; and netiquette. Breaches in any of these categories can result in a range of outcomes from minor repercussions through loss of respect by peers to loss of licensure and employment. Some breaches can carry legal liability: sexual boundary violations; lack of confidentiality of patient information; inadvertently creating a treatment relationship; not meeting the required standard of care; and practicing medicine without a license.

As outlined in Chapter 11, standards are emerging around the use of social media and digital technology in healthcare, and professionals working in health care need to be aware of these. Professional organizations, licensing boards, health-care institutions, and malpractice insurers may all have their own specific standards.

However, as we saw in Chapter 12, technology in health care is changing constantly and rapidly. How can health-care professionals stay current in terms of professional practices and standards using social media and the Internet? How can we as a field both take advantage of all that technology has to offer health care without compromising our professionalism?

First, we must keep talking about these issues. Professional workshops and meetings can serve as a forum to discuss current practices and concerns about them. Generational differences need to be respected, and a nonjudgmental approach assumed. Otherwise, the risk is that clinicians will go "underground" with their digital behavior, and exacerbate an already reported trend in medical ethics – that health-care professionals say one thing and do another.

Second, we must teach about professionalism and technology to trainees entering health-care professions. Digital natives, for whom boundaries of privacy and intellectual property have been redefined and for whom the Internet is an extension of themselves, may be completely unaware of some of the professionalism issues associated with the use of digital media. They need to be explicitly taught.

Real-life examples provide excellent teaching tools. Peer supervision around how to manage technological dilemmas as they present can provide a protected forum for discussion of these issues. The AADPRT Curriculum on Professionalism and the Internet offers one teaching model.

When I started thinking about professionalism and the Internet, I focused on online behaviors and breaches of professionalism standards.

What has become clear, however, is that while professional use of technology can be demonstrated using clinical vignettes, these vignettes about digital technology also serve as an excellent way to teach about professionalism. Thus, behavior on the Internet and social media is a microcosm for overall professional behavior in health care. By using examples pertaining to digital media in our teaching, we may capture the millennial generation and have an opportunity to make professionalism seem relevant and important.

Why is professional use of social media and the Internet so important in health care? As discussed in Chapter 1, part of the answer lies in the importance of trust in the treatment relationship, both on an individual level between treaters and their patients, and between the health-care professional and society in general. The importance of maintaining that trust cannot be overstated.

Equally important, however, is that how we as a profession manage social media and the Internet *now* may have prognostic value for the *future*. Inevitably, more and more information will become available through technology, and some of that data is highly sensitive. Recall the MIT scientists who discovered the identities of anonymous DNA donors to research projects via simple online technologies. Genetic and "personalized" treatments for common disorders such as cancer are increasingly available in health care, and this information will of necessity be stored in electronic medical records. The use of "big data," aggregating information from multiple sources, is likely to increase in health care.

Similarly, technology itself is likely to become more powerful and sophisticated. Leaping into the newest technologies may become increasingly risky in terms of the potential for errors, with significant consequences for patient wellbeing and professionalism. Establishing professional patterns of behavior around technology use and learning how to acquire knowledge and skill as new technologic capacities develop are vital.

Thus, as the digital revolution unavoidably further disrupts health care, the stakes appear to be increasing. The importance of health-care professionals demonstrating respect for boundaries, privacy, confidentiality, and other tenets of professionalism is and will be extraordinarily high. If we cannot find a way to manage digital technology professionally today, we may not be prepared for the brave new world of tomorrow.

Index

Printed and bound by CPI Group (UK) Ltd, Croydon, CR0 4YY

03/10/2024

01040423-0018